The Air That I Breathe

Hope and Healing from Anxiety

22 Day and Night Devotions

Jodi Howe

Copyright

© 1968 Helen Steiner Rice Foundation Fund, LLC
a wholly owned subsidiary of
Cincinnati Museum Center

Scripture taken from the New King James Version®. Copyright © 1982 by Thomas Nelson. Used by permission. All rights reserved.

Scripture quotations marked (NIV) are taken from the Holy Bible, New International Version®, NIV®. Copyright © 1973, 1978, 1984, 2011 by Biblica, Inc.™ Used by permission of Zondervan. All rights reserved worldwide. www.zondervan.com The "NIV" and "New International Version" are trademarks registered in the United States Patent and Trademark Office by Biblica, Inc.™

A Note from Jodi

Thank you, God. With gratitude I write this. In prayer, I hope it helps others. In faith, I trust it will. In love, I honor You with my words.

"When you begin to breathe the air of Jesus, His spirit lives within you, offering hope and peace as a testimony to His love!" -Jodi Howe

God sent His Son to the cross, introduced me to Jesus, and took my secular breathe away. He gave me new spiritual air to breathe in filled with faith, hope, trust, and love.

God gave me a peaceful mind. This peace became a peace that surpasses all understanding.

I want that for you.

I believe God does too.

His Word tells us, "Do not worry, do not be anxious, do not fear" hundreds of times in the Bible. That's the truth, and anxiety is well under His control too. The secret is that we must seek Him for that peace. It's simpler than you think.

That's what this book is about.

I will guide you.

God will order your steps. Here is how I know.

I have suffered from anxiety and panic disorder for decades.

I first experienced anxiety when I was young, heading to my college graduation. Subsequently, it reappeared throughout my adult life. During a time when it was more stigmatic, I had fewer opportunities to understand it, embrace it, or heal from it. But God has a way.

The Air That I Breathe

It wasn't until a cold winter in 2009 that I hit a mental rock bottom–for no reason. There was no trauma, hardship, or death; life seemed good. But spiritually, to my dismay, I was a wreck. And I didn't even know it. Yet God did.

The Lord needed to reach me so I could fulfill my future mission(s). He knew I was too hardheaded to seek Him naturally. He saw me selfishly living for the world. I was selfishly living for myself. God knew in order to lift me, He had to bring me to my knees. Through this season of rebirth, I was redeemed and renewed.

Anxiety comes in many forms. General fear. Constant worry. A mental (medical) illness. PTSD and Trauma. And all fall under a worldly cause with a hopeful result in healing. And for me, a calling to share the "good news."

I am here to tell you that they are healable through effort. It starts with discovering the actual reasons why you may be anxious. I'll get to that in this book.

There is one false claim I want to uncover first so we can heal properly. I discovered an approach to anxiety in the Christian faith that suggests if you "pray it away, it will go away." My pain is your gain and I want to save you some time. I am here to shut that down right now.

Yes, it is a style of belief that people fall prey to, including myself. I believed that by praying to God and waiting to be healed with a quick prayer of one, two, and three, I could rub the genie, which would be enough. Then, I learned this life-changing fact. It takes actual work to grow toward healing.

As stated in this book, the concept of "pray it away" is not sustainable for healing from anxiety. This perspective challenged me the most. But God is the God of clarity. And wow, do I get it now!

You may be unconscious of your anxious reality. For some, you live with it without realizing it. It's okay; I did too. That is why you are here

Jodi Howe

reading this. So stick with me and give me the benefit of the doubt so you can learn a new perspective.

You do have the ability to aid in the prosperity of your spirit, soul, and body. By applying physical or medicinal aids towards healing your body, in addition to prayer and your walk with Christ, God will move this anxious mountain standing right in front of you.

It's important to mention that my upbringing was not under a biblical Christian doctrine. Though I was raised in the church under the Catholic faith, I never had a relationship with Jesus. I was a Chr-easter. In other words, I showed up to Christmas and Easter services.

Under my mother's strong faith, I heard that God is a massive power in life and can perform miracles. Yet it wasn't until I became mentally ill that I learned that relationship building with Jesus is where the foundation of real peace comes from, where joy resides, and where pain goes the wayside.

There is tremendous power in prayer. But we have a spirit, soul, and body. They all need to do their due diligence.

I have always approached the role of God as the almighty, yet common sense taught me that I still had to put my two feet forward to follow His lead. In other words, yes, He can do the supernatural in your life, but you must still do your part. Worthy is anyone who is open to direction, faith, and trust.

I hope to help ease you through this difficult time while you attempt to heal your anxiety. Yet, in good faith, I feel led to introduce you to Jesus first and foremost. If Jesus hasn›t already entered your heart, would you consider a relationship with Him? No worries if you're not there right now. A journey in faith is a marathon, not a sprint. Take heart, Jesus overcame the world, and when you walk with Him, He will take you under His mighty control.

The Air That I Breathe

Jesus only wants to know you more and see you prosper through His promises. In Colossians 3:15, Paul tells us, "And let the peace of God rule in your hearts, to which also you were called in one body; And be thankful."

When Jesus is in our hearts, there is an inevitable peace through storms. It may be hard to understand initially, but if you are willing, allow His grace to unfold in you! And let my testimony and "tried and true tips" aid in your healing.

To others who are in sync with the Holy Spirit, may you continually call upon Jesus during your times of fear, confusion, and anxiety.

In addition to a relationship with Jesus, God wants us to be proactive in maintaining our best selves and respecting our bodies while striving for good health.

Yet God does not want you to do this alone.

He provides his earth with medicine, doctors, healthcare, churches, fellowships, small groups, family, friends, communities, and so much more. Embrace them all, or just start with one. If you take this leap of faith, I am confident you will find support for this life challenge.

Worship Song Suggestion:
MAKE ROOM
By, The Church Will Sing,
Elyssa Smith,
Community Music

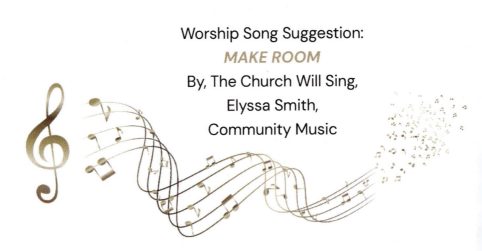

My Testimony

I was walking through my college graduation at Syracuse University, not knowing what was happening to my mind and body. Out of nowhere, I started to sweat, feel faint, and the world felt like it was closing in on me.

I had to leave the processional and was led to the Carrier Dome's medic room to live out four hours of my college finale instead of celebrating four years' worth of an earned graduation day, because my mind was telling me I was experiencing a heart attack. Instead, I learned I was having an anxiety attack. And the milestone was over.

The medics did a full workup and released me, assuring me I was okay. To this day, I believe my mother still thinks I overslept and missed my graduation. I moved on.

Fast-forward months later, another anxiety attack hit while I was out with friends. This brought me to the emergency room, still not understanding what was happening to my body. An EKG and full workup with healthy results assured the doctors I was okay. I moved on.

Several years later, I lived in northern California with my soon-to-be husband. He traveled a lot, and I was left alone. That brought loneliness that turned into fear of the future, which resulted in a third anxiety attack.

At this point, the internet was available, and although we didn't have a minuscule of what we have in terms of research now, it was still a source of information. I researched my symptoms and discovered I have anxiety and panic disorder. Wait a minute; do I have a mental illness?

Yet at the time, mental illness carried a huge stigma, spurring feelings that made me feel like a "crazy" person. I honestly didn't know where

The Air That I Breathe

to turn. I talked to a doctor, and he tried giving me some strategies to work through it, which I believe helped in the short term. He assured me I was just fine. The symptoms, they subsided. I moved on.

Life played its lovely course and faithfully brought me to married life and children. A move back to the East Coast and back to family roots brought a new life. It seemed my anxiety disorder was gone. I didn't even think much about it. Then, the year before I turned forty, my anxiety and panic disorder returned with a vengeance. Besides the fear of getting older, I didn't have specific reasons for feeling anxious. But I was terrified. There were never specific reasons, just reasons that manifested in my mind. Since then, I have learned I was suffering from a chemical and hormonal imbalance, which led to a complete loss of control of my mind.

This episode was so severe that I physically got sick. I couldn't eat, I couldn't sleep, and I couldn't function. And this time my doctor couldn't "in good faith" or good practice assure me I was just fine. And in no way, shape, or form could I move on.

After much research, I decided Western medicine was necessary to regain my life. In addition, I began to shift my thought process with a radical acceptance that this was my cross to bear. Even though I was still underwater and needed to continue fighting through this storm, as the waves subsided, I found a different kind of medicine, a raft, that changed my life forever.

As I struggled to survive, my mother was very concerned and, like many, lacked knowledge in this area. She would pray and worry and pray some more.

One day, my mother came to my home and told me to see a devout Christian friend. I thought that was weird and illogical. Denise was a family friend we had known for years. She was close to my mother as they had worked together during my adolescence, but to me she was a random family friend I saw occasionally. We had no relationship, and the thought of visiting her didn't help my anxiety. However, my mother relentlessly insisted I reach out to her. I took a leap of faith to avoid disappointing her.

I contacted Denise and decided to meet at her home for lunch. When I arrived, she had just gotten off the phone with her sister Katherine. Katherine lived in England and was on her deathbed, suffering from various physical diseases. But through it all, she loved, praised, and worshiped Christ in her every-waking moment.

Denise told me they were praying for me before my arrival. I was not a believer, so this was odd and, quite frankly, made me uncomfortable. But I followed through with my mother's plea for this meeting and let the cards fall as they would.

Denise and I talked awhile about life and anxiety, and she asked if she could pray with me. I said yes, and after that, she asked if I would be willing to join a Bible study with her. My initial quiet thought was, heck no. I don't do Bible studies. But to be considerate, I told her I would think about it.

The thought of a Bible study was awkward and, quite frankly, seemed like a waste of my time.

After I left her home, I felt so many things. Emotions tugged at my heartstrings. Yet there was a hint of inspiration floating through my soul.

I was raised Catholic and had heard of Jesus through that doctrine. However, I did not have a relationship with Him. In fact, for over thirty years, I walked into these tremendous, beautiful stain-glassed cathedral foundations, and there He was, hanging on the cross for all eyes to witness. Jesus. He was right there! Yet, I had no idea who He was.

I accepted her invitation, and my mother and I attended our first Bible study.

The Air That I Breathe

I knew very little of the Bible except for bits and pieces, like the story of Adam and Eve. I also recognized Moses from a Hollywood film and learned parts of the Gospels from playing Mary of Magdalene in Jesus Christ Superstar; needless to say, I was clueless.

The Bible can be intimidating! And like others who were in the infant stages of learning, I was overwhelmed and felt foolish.

Denise chose a study that was a great starting point–introducing the Bible and faith in a 101-style format.

I stayed committed. As the weeks flew by, I began to know Jesus. I was intrigued and thought about Him increasingly, putting Him at the forefront of my thinking. And, like some, I had an aha moment when I was driving home from a store. This is the first time Jesus spoke to me.

Being an avid lover of music and devoting my life to singing, it's not surprising that Jesus would choose this forum to speak to me. Like most people, I had many songs on my phone's playlist. Songs that mainly spoke to a secular worldview. Yet I did have two Christian songs.

"There is a God," by Lee Ann Womack.

"I Can Only Imagine," by Mercy Me.

I was having a hard day. The healing process from anxiety was not an overnight quick fix. After leaving the store, I got into my car, pushed the random button on my playlist, and out of hundreds of songs, those two played one after the other.

Christ leaped into my soul, and I was born again in Him!

I wrote this book to honor God. Although He has been my heavenly Father my whole life, I now see how He began "showing up" due to my anxiety. I can proclaim that He saved me, that I was reborn, breathing new air and seeing life through a different lens. There is a unique perspective, daily hope, and trust that anxiety will never take over my life again. And it hasn't.

I was able to form a relationship with Jesus that grows daily. And through that growth, I see Him working in my life, strengthening it from every angle, including anxiety, relationships, children, and endless blessings.

Some may already know this relationship and flex the Holy Spirit of Jesus daily. To others who are not actively following Jesus, that's okay too; I was you.

It was anxiety disorder that brought me to Christ. He works in mysterious and beautiful ways, and your first effort to open this book may be your lighthouse to the ultimate peace only Jesus can provide.

Pastor and Bible commentator Alexander Maclaren said, "Peace is not the absence of problems, it's the presence of God!"

Throughout my journey with Christ and writing this book, I received resistance from naysayers telling me I may not understand anxiety well enough to share it with the intent to aid in healing. I also learned that this world sees anxiety differently. There are many aspects of anxiety! When someone says they are dealing with anxiety, it's essential to understand what type they are dealing with.

My anxiety falls under general anxiety and panic disorder, a treatable mental illness. But as I researched other forms, I generally found that most (or all) are suffering from general anxiety disorder. Some live daily under what they believe to be normal or acceptable forms of anxiety without understanding it. Regardless of what form of anxiety yours falls under, all of this information is applicable.

In writing this, I hope to encourage you to trust in the Lord and apply practical measures to help you feel less or no anxiety so you can live the best life God wants for you.

Are you longing for a peaceful mind? Do you suffer from anxiety and panic disorder?

The Air That I Breathe

Trusting God through the storms in your mind can work wonders.

Jesus is the pillar of wonders overcoming the world. Trusting in Him brought about miracles that began to unfold before my eyes.

Now, onto the more "medical" questions.

Do you know the difference between a panic attack and other severe, anxiety-related health issues?

Have you:

Told your doctor about your symptoms?

- Started a new therapy regimen?
- Started exercising or taking simple brisk walks?
- Changed your diet and considered avoiding things that can cause anxiety?

Maybe you have decided to start medication. Yes, it's a lot to take in.

There are many ways to ease daily anxiety, yet take note: You need not suffer any longer than you already have. Through the strength of the Lord, fellowship, supportive doctors, and the ultimate decision to include medication, I am a healed testimony to that.

It will take a little time. But give yourself grace. You've opened up this book and chosen to accept your current state.

Your willingness to put in the work is a significant next step. You are embracing clearing your mind and seeking a peaceful center.

God promises you will get there. Why? Because He offers thousands of promises in the Bible of how much He loves us and wants us to find freedom and peace in Him.

Just stay focused on Jesus, and He will lead the way. He will never let you down. I know this because He's never let me down.

So what can I offer you?

In this book, I will offer you tips. Tried and true methods of healing anxiety. Some have been around for centuries; others are new discoveries. I have tried them all, and they work.

I am not a doctor, nor will I pretend to be one here. I encourage you to be under the advisement of a medical doctor or therapist to aid in this journey.

In this daily format, I offer the ability to take each day and night step by step to avoid feeling overwhelmed. But, if you want to go ahead a day or two, go for it. As I began my healing journey, I discovered it was hard to get up in the morning and face the day in fear of anxious thoughts and panic attacks. Whether it's mental illness that adds to daily fear or other aspects encouraging anxiety, you must approach it from many different angles. Don't worry; I will cover those angles.

While the beginning of the day was hard, going to bed at night offered its own set of worries. I had trouble falling asleep and staying asleep, because I feared more panic attacks would awaken me. At night, panic attacks are more controlling and can produce more intense fear. I will cover this, too.

Because I speak to Christians, I will talk from a doctrinal perspective. Therefore, I encourage you to start and end each day in Scripture before you try anything. Then prayer.

The Bible is my daily hope. When I began highlighting His promises by finding God-breathed words relating to this kind of suffering, God gave me endurance and prompted me to share this wisdom with you.

My prayer is that you:

- Find your daily hope in Jesus.
- Start healing from anxiety.
- Begin to feel peace that surpasses all understanding.

The Air That I Breathe

God is a good, good father, and He loves you so much. Let's pray for a new beginning in healing anxiety by allowing God to release the chains that bind us in fear.

Dear Father God,

I begin this pathway to healing by trusting You. Please hold my hand through the fear. Walk beside me through the hurt. Lift me when worry weighs me down. I will start my days with You. Please send me those gentle reminders with each new light.

In Jesus's name, amen.

Worship Song Suggestion:
BELIEVE FOR IT
By, CeCe Winans
and
Worship Song Suggestion:
ALWAYS THERE
By, Natalie Grant

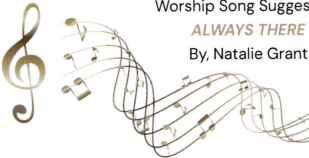

Jodi Howe

Day 1

I know it's hard to believe that the supernatural gift of faith, hope, and love can get you from a place of panic to peace. I completely get it because I was you. But I took that leap of faith a decade later; I can honestly say it was God. It is God. And it will forever be God's grace that has healed me from anxiety. So, if you're willing, please give me the benefit of the doubt and keep reading.

I know that He will never abandon nor forsake you. Especially now, when you need Him the most.

Tip of the day: Take a leap of faith

The LORD will give strength to His people; the LORD will bless His people with peace. Psalms 29:11 NKJV

Praying and being still are critical to getting the spirit, soul, and body on track. Even if you rush out to work in the morning, do your best to allow yourself five to ten minutes of prayer and focus time on the Lord. Five minutes with Him can surprise you with twenty-three hours and fifty-five minutes of peace, strength, and endurance for anything that comes your way.

Sometimes, getting out of bed and dealing with your day is challenging when you are in storms of anxious episodes. The fear of being generally anxious all day, having a panic attack (or several), and not having control of your thoughts can be debilitating. Those fears take over, and it's hard to feel positive that a new day could give you a renewed sense of hope that your therapy and medication (if you choose to take it) are working.

But God is working to heal you and bring you closer to Him. Stay focused on Him and on track with your efforts to begin the process of healing. Even though you can't see Him, know that through the Holy Spirit, He is there and has never and will never leave your side.

Dear Lord,

I am taking this leap of faith today, knowing you are walking alongside me with every step. Please remind me to call upon you when I feel out of control and scared. I cannot deliver myself from fear, but You can, and with that, I feel more at peace. Thank You.

In Jesus's name, amen.

Jodi Howe

Take Aways:

Action Steps:

Night 1

I remember believing that there was no way this anxiety would ever go away. I remember having nights of ultimate fear and panic that this was my new life and I would always live in this pain. But take heart. Not only did Jesus overcome the world, but He also renewed me and helped me to overcome anxiety. I just had to work to get to where I am today. By His grace, of course!

 Tip of the night: This too shall pass!

Then Jesus spoke to them again, saying, "I am the light of the world. He who follows Me shall not walk in darkness but have the light of life." John 8:12 NKJV

Have a backup plan if you have trouble sleeping. It's essential to avoid tossing and turning for hours on end. You will not be able to get your body back to sleep, and lack of sleep encourages more stress, which brings on anxiety.

Rest assured, if you walk with Him, the darkness will fade. If you have moments where you wake up with panic, immediately call upon the Lord and ask Him to calm your mind and spirit, and He will wrap you in a blanket of peace. Doctors say that if you have times in the middle of the night when you're tossing and turning and unable to sleep, get out of bed, go to another dimly lit location, and read for about ten to twenty minutes. That should bring you to a drowsy state, and then once you feel sleepy again, go back into bed and try to sleep. Of course, I only read positive, inspirational, and motivating things. A beneficial book I suggest is, you guessed it, the Bible. The book of Job is a powerful story of life, loss, and life renewed. In the book of Psalms, amidst his trials and doubts, David reveres the Lord. Also, the Gospels are filled with acclamations of Jesus's last days on earth.

Research some great Christian authors who have written faith-based books that help bring you closer to the Word through testimony and inspiration.

We all struggle, and our testimonies reassure the world that God is real and is the God of redemption.

Before I came to Christ, I was intrigued by a writer named Helen Steiner Rice. My mother had given me a book over thirty years ago that I have to this day. I now see how God was knocking at my door even then. I used to be drawn to these devotionals even before I knew Jesus Christ and had accepted a relationship with Him. They truly did help me through some challenging times. How often I needed these books during the darkest moments of my life, only to find peace at the end!

The following is from one of Helen Steiner Rice's books. I think you may benefit from reading it. It was a lifeline for me. I prayed it over and over.

This Too Shall Pass.

This Too Shall Pass

If I can endure for this minute
Whatever is happening to me,
No matter how heavy my heart is
Or how dark the moment may be–

If I can remain calm and quiet
With all the world crashing about me,
Secure in the knowledge God loves me
When everyone else seems to doubt me–

If I can but keep on believing
What I know in my heart to be true,
That darkness will fade with the morning
And this will pass away, too–

Then nothing in life can defeat me
For as long as this knowledge remains
I can suffer whatever is happening
For I know God will break all the chains

That are binding me tight in the darkness
And trying to fill me with fear–
There is no night without dawning
And I know my morning is near.

Helen Steiner Rice[1]

---

[1] Reprinted with permission of the Helen Steiner Rice Foundation Fund, LLC

Jodi Howe

Father God and Light of the World, lead me out of the darkness. Develop, within me, the confidence that a new day will dawn and with it new hope.

Amen!

I pray this brings you hope tonight.

Worship Song Suggestion:
RESCUE
By, Jason Ingram

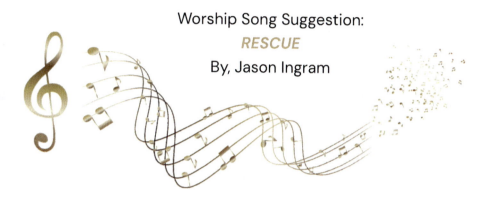

Take Aways:

Action Steps:

Day 2

*I*was under a doctor's care as this anxiety spiraled out of control. He kept mentioning medicine, and I was very reluctant. I tried everything under the sun—ate healthily, had no caffeine or alcohol, and exercised, used lavender, went to therapy, and practiced faith-based meditation.

And all of those were helpful. But only partially sustainable in the long term.

That's how bad this anxiety was.

It was when I submitted to the expertise of my physician, embraced my reality, and ultimately started a faith walk that the true healing began.

Tip of the day: Doctor, doctor. Give me the news ...

If any of you lacks wisdom, let him ask of God, who gives to all liberally and without reproach, and it will be given him. James 1:5 NKJV

Call your doctor. There may be underlying issues as to why you are anxious. Complete physical health is necessary for your peace of mind so you can begin healing.

The wisdom of God is our best hope. He gives us good reasons and vessels to find such knowledge to journey through life. Do not disregard your anxiety. It is a disease; like all diseases, it needs a doctor's diagnosis and healing. See a doctor for a complete physical, especially for the correct diagnosis and the peace of mind that nothing more profound or underlying is occurring in your body. Many diseases and ailments instigate anxiety, and you must rule anything and everything out. If there

The Air That I Breathe

are no underlying causes, your anxiety will heal knowing you're in better health than you thought. But if there are underlying problems, getting down to the root of it can be peace enough.

Father God,

I seek Your wisdom always and during this struggle, I need it. Bring me to the proper physician who leads with understanding and good practice to assist in my healing.

It's in Jesus's name, amen.

Take Aways:

Action Steps:

Night 2

I was so afraid to consider any Western medicine assistance in healing my anxiety. I was worried I'd be labeled a freak and that there would be many side effects. But I didn't have the facts, just influences from the world and Dr. Google. It wasn't until I started a therapy regimen that I could focus on the more essential things, such as getting better physically and mentally. It allowed me to function so my mind could open up to what God was doing in my life.

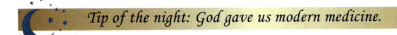

Tip of the night: God gave us modern medicine.

And when Jesus went out He saw a great multitude, and He was moved with compassion for them and healed their sick. Matthew 14:14 NKJV

There are millions of people every day who are afraid to take medicine. Even if the medication is *for anxiety*, some people are too anxious to take it! (I, too, felt this way.)

Understanding anxiety teaches you what causes these fears and what you can do about them.

Our mind can tend to be our worst enemy in telling us foolish thoughts, such as, "If we take anxiety medicines, we are now labeled "crazy" or "can't control our minds." Or other things that our mind taunts us with. If you had diabetes, would you deny yourself insulin? If you had cancer and your only hope was chemotherapy, would you decline it? For most, the answer is no.

As you talk to your doctor about options, use your prayer time, wise mind, and the trusted one who went to medical school to help you make the best choice for your healing.

Jodi Howe

Dear Father,

I am tortured by the mental games I play with myself in resisting options for healing. Those fears do not aid in the recovery of my anxiety. You know what's best for my body, and I fervently pray that you guide me in making the best choices possible. If medicine is the best option right now, please impart knowledge, wisdom, and trust in my heart, assuring me this is within Your plan. I am hanging on with the grace of Your Son, Jesus.

I pray this to You, amen

Worship Song Suggestion:
WAYMAKER
By, Michael W. Smith

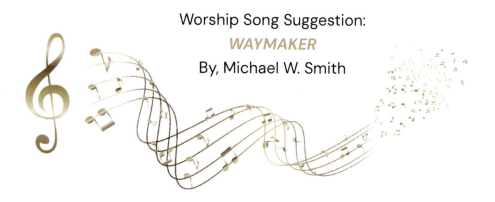

Take Aways:

Action Steps:

Jodi Howe

Day 3

You have to be very careful about what you put into your body while trying to control your anxiety. I had to avoid caffeine or anything that instigated my anxiety. I stopped coffee altogether. I didn't drink any alcohol or anything else that would stimulate my body. I also abstained from eating heavy, greasy foods or foods containing abundant sugars and processed ingredients. It was helpful.

Ironically, as I have control over my anxiety today, I still follow a very similar diet regimen, with an occasional celebration of tasty foods and drinks here or there.

And the Lord knows I need my coffee.

 Tip of the day: Don't instigate your anxiety!

Therefore, whether you eat or drink, or whatever you do, do all to the glory of God. 1 Corinthians 10:31 NKJV

Avoid caffeine and other stimulants incredibly late in the day. It agitates the mind and works to encourage *more* anxiety.

Caffeine, energy drinks, nicotine—I suggest you avoid them.

I love coffee! But as I worked to heal from my anxiety, I avoided caffeine until I gained control over my anxious circumstances. So, in due time, you can have that glorious cup of Joe in the morning. But for now, get your energy from natural ingredients, healthy morning fruit and protein shakes, or even a brisk walk.

Avoid anything with heavy amounts of caffeine, like energy drinks. I'll never encourage them because they're unhealthy for you, period!

The Air That I Breathe

Dear Lord,

I fervently ask You right now to control my mind. My overwhelming, wandering thoughts of worry and fear are crippling me. I so desperately need Your peace and assurance that I will heal. I have chosen to come to You, but it's in Your grace that You are always with me. I may need gentle reminders occasionally, but I ask that You show up and start Your healing today. Thank You for Your wisdom.

In Jesus's beautiful name. amen.

Take Aways:

Action Steps:

Night 3

Growing up, the only prayer I ever knew was the childhood one that most know as, "Now I lay me down to sleep …"

Praying was so foreign to me as I started this walk. I felt intimidated by others who pray fluently and beautifully. It can make you feel like an idiot when you open your mouth and talk to God. I know how that feels. But God doesn't care about pretty prayers. He wants to hear from us and commune with our hearts. Scripture tells us to give our requests to God. So, if we pray for healing and peace, He will hear and provide. All you have to do is start the conversation!

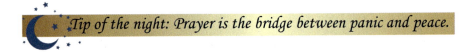

Tip of the night: Prayer is the bridge between panic and peace.

Fear not, for I am with you; Be not dismayed, for I am your God. I will strengthen you, I will also help you, I will uphold you with My righteous right hand. Isaiah 41:10 NKJV

The promise is right there. Our heavenly Father *will* help you. And how do we seek help? We pray.

Prayer strengthens us. It takes us out of our heads and into connection with God. It's how we give Him our worries and how He speaks to us. It gets transmitted through the Holy Spirit, the gift of God's presence that Jesus left for us.

Anxiety is debilitating and can affect our life's potential or daily function.

Sometimes, the night can get scary and overwhelming. Living in constant fear is no way to live. Jesus does not want you to suffer, and God is not the God of fear.

Jodi Howe

If you open your heart and mind to Jesus, He will be the presence of hope to you through the Holy Spirit.

He's got your anxiety right under His righteous hand. If you are willing to trust and follow Him.

Jesus is such a great friend and listener. I encourage you to get to know Him more. He doesn't talk back to us like our kids do. He is so gracious.

Dear Lord,

I made it through the day. Now, I yearn for a peaceful sleep. I know it takes time to control my anxiety fully, but I ask that You give me a calm approach to my nighttime and ease my mind into beautiful thoughts that only You and Your miraculous power can provide. I am grateful to get to know You more.

In your Son's glorious name, amen.

Worship Song Suggestion:
YOU'RE GONNA BE OKAY
By, Brian and Jenn Johnson

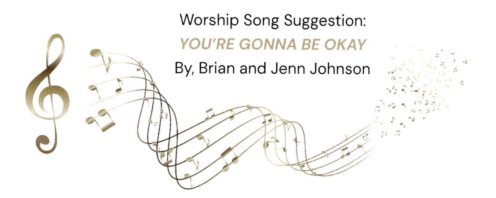

Take Aways:

Action Steps:

Jodi Howe

Day 4

*E*ducate yourself! The more I learned about anxiety and its associated effects, the more knowledge I gained about what I should and shouldn't do to get healthy. And I know that immediately running to the internet is a double-edged sword. So be wary of what you find from non-credible people and where you seek information.

 Tip of the day: "A" is for anxiety.

The heart of the prudent acquires knowledge, And the ear of the wise seeks knowledge. Proverbs 18:15 NKJV

It's essential to know anxiety's cause and effect. Knowledge makes you more aware of the triggers and can aid you with successful coping mechanisms. This could be a matter of life or that dreaded feeling of death your mind creates.

Be careful of Dr. Google! It can send you into an immense panic. Choose your sources wisely. Learn the facts and find references to manage your daily life. I recommend The Anxiety & Phobia Workbook (latest edition) by Edmund J. Bourne, PhD. There are also some fabulous podcasts out there. I suggest listening to those who genuinely understand anxiety as testimony or are clinically educated. But I will most especially encourage you to have this conversation with your physician.

Father,

As I dive into this disease, I am more grateful for Your love, support, and grace that will inevitably bring me to a place of daily peace and hope that I can live with anxiety and still prosper abundantly with You by my side. In Jesus's name, amen.

The Air That I Breathe

Take Aways:

Action Steps:

Night 4

*I*t is best to recognize this: life is full of trials and pain. Jesus said, "Take heart, I have overcome the world, so I can overcome any problem that afflicted you" (John 16:33 my paraphrase).

There's probably very little you can do under your mortal cognition. Worry is truly not trusting in God. It is a waste of energy. I learned that it's not worth our time because it can make us physically sick and drain precious time that God wants us to embrace.

 Tip of the night: ♪ *Don't worry, be holy.* ♪

Therefore, do not worry about tomorrow, for tomorrow will worry about its own things. Sufficient for the day is its own trouble. Matthew 6:34 NKJV

I find such solace in the above Scripture as this chapter discusses time wasted (and inevitably ineffective) when leading with worry. Worry is a part of anxiety. Whether you have a general anxiety disorder or situational anxiety, it's the enemy rearing his ugly head trying to elevate your state of mind, which hinders your healing.

Take heart and journal the positive and joyful events, activities, and actions your tomorrow can and will hold. You are in control of more than your mind lets you believe. A simple prayer to Jesus is impactful.

The Air That I Breathe

Dear Lord,

My anxious thoughts get the better of me every day. Please instill in me the ability to rely on Your miraculous ways of turning worry into wonder. Remind me that I can prosper with positivity and peace. You are joy. So in You, I find joy. Life is filled with troubles, but why should I worry if I have You leading my day?

It's in your Son's name, I pray, amen!

Worship Song Suggestion:
JOY IN THE MORNING
By, Tauren Wells,
Elevation Worship

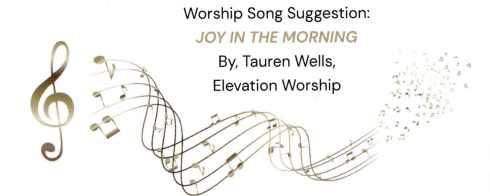

Jodi Howe

Take Aways:

Action Steps:

Day 5

I am a worship leader. I've been singing my entire life and have been blessed to be under excellent voice coaching. The breathing that I speak of in this book is the same breathing training that I give my voice students. I am thrilled that I can share it so that it will help you. And if you have a singing voice, apply this because it works.

 Tip of the day: The air that I breathe.

The Spirit of God has made me, and the breathe of the Almighty gives me life. Job 33:4 NKJV

Practice deep breathing from the diaphragm rather than the chest. This is a great way to relax and reduce anxiety. Although we should all breathe this way, very few do so. Practice this breathing pattern while you are in a relaxed and safe environment. This way, you will be more likely to use this technique when faced with situations that trigger the symptoms of anxiety or a panic attack.

When you suffer from anxiety and panic attacks, it's essential to have a strategy in place. Breathing is a great way to help reset yourself and take you out of that fight or flight response, especially if you're feeling extreme anxiety or you sense panic attacks coming on. There's nothing wrong with removing yourself from any situation, going to a quiet place, and just remembering to breathe.

1. Find a quiet place free of distractions. Lie somewhere or recline in a chair, loosen any tight clothing, and remove obstacles. Rest your hands in your lap or on the arms of the chair.
2. Place one hand on your upper chest and the other on your stomach. Inhale, taking a deep breathe from your abdomen as you count to

five. As you inhale, you should feel your belly rise. The hand on your chest should not move.
3. After a short pause, slowly exhale while counting to five. Your stomach should fall back down as you exhale.
4. Continue this pattern of rhythmic breathing for five to ten minutes.

Father God,

I ask You to come into my day and keep me out of any situations that may cause fear. Anxiety brings me extreme fight and flight thoughts, and I don't want that in my day. I want to have You in my day, all day, and let You be "the air that I breathe."

It's in Jesus's beautiful name, amen.

Take Aways:

Action Steps:

Jodi Howe

Night 5

God reminded us that on the seventh day, we are to rest. You need to rest at some point throughout the day. And if you can make your nighttime routine a place of relaxation, your sleep will become blissful too. Friends, I am a stickler about this. My sleep is most important to me, and the prep beforehand is pretty detailed, much like a spa retreat. And in case you're interested, my favorite scent is lavender.

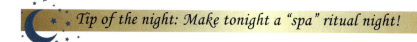
Tip of the night: Make tonight a "spa" ritual night!

I will both lie down in peace, and sleep; For You alone, O Lord, make me dwell in safety. Psalms 4:8 NKJV

End your day with a long, relaxing bath or shower. It truly allows you to refresh and calm your mind, allowing your body to return to a relaxed state. Light candles, play soft music, and take some "you" time. Self-care is essential for you to tend to those around you the next day.

Add some aromatherapy like lavender, vanilla, eucalyptus, mint, ginger, orange, lemon, rosemary, jasmine, or sandalwood. They reduce anxiety and are oh, so lovely.

Top it off with aromatherapy lotions, comfy pajamas, and praise music, singing to the Lord. Tell Him that you appreciate His mighty presence in your life.

Lord knows I do.

The Air That I Breathe

Dear Father,

As I enter what I hope to be a peaceful slumber, I ask that You stay with me. As I continue the healing process of my anxiety, I know there may be moments when I feel scared. Moments that might wake me up and bring me to a place of panic. I fervently ask You to calm those fears and return me to a beautiful sleep. You are allowing me to wake up in the morning. So with extreme gratitude, I thank You for Your loyalty and grace.

In Jesus's beautiful name, amen.

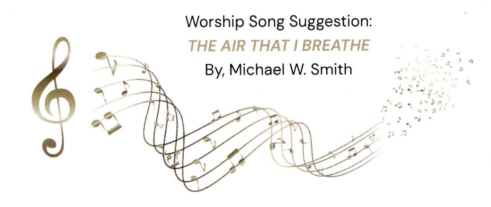

Worship Song Suggestion:
THE AIR THAT I BREATHE
By, Michael W. Smith

Take Aways:

Action Steps:

The Air That I Breathe

Day 6

I can't stress this enough: giving your time to the Lord can change your day. And then your life. I have learned that this is a critical lesson in any form of growth in our spirit. It's a no-brainer and a game-changer.

You can't win at the game of life if you aren't in the Book of Life.

 Tip of the day: Give your first five minutes to God.

> *Until now you have asked nothing in My name. Ask, and you will receive, that your joy may be full. John 16:24 NKJV*

Even if you have a busy life where you wake up to the chaos of raising kids, meeting school demands, or getting ready for work, do your best to find time to read a devotional. You may need to wake up early before the family in order to make time. Consider reading a Scripture, practicing breathing, listening to light worship music, and praying.

His promises are grand. His mercy is plentiful. His grace is sufficient. His love is powerful.

He watches over us with every walk and breathe we take. Be sure to start your day with Him in the forefront of everything you do so you can see His grace and blessings with every occurrence, good or not-so-good.

Father God,

As I walk through this day, I ask that You walk with me, keeping my mind focused on You and Your glory. Grant me the grace I need to act and react as Jesus would. If I falter and fear creeps in, remind me to tell the enemy he is not allowed in my day, my thoughts, my world, "in Jesus's name"! I know instantly that Your light will start to shine.

Always in Your beautiful name, amen.

Night 6

*M*y growth in ministry came through my willingness to study. I sought Scriptures that spoke to anxiety, which moved me towards healing. I found Bible verses that answered my fears with promises of peace, and it allowed me to build endurance through anxiety (and in life in general).

I am a crazy notetaker, a journal girl, and most significantly, I have so much content that I don't even know what to do with it. Or do I? That's where this book right here started. Also, I created a podcast to encourage a deeper relationship with Christ. It's called The Air That I Breathe.

Tip of the night: Jot it down!

Then He said to His disciples, "Therefore I say to you, do not worry about your life, what you will eat; nor about the body, what you will put on. Life is more than food and the body is more than clothing. Consider the ravens, for they neither sow nor reap, which have neither storehouse nor barn; and God feeds them. Of how much more value are you than the birds? And which of you by worrying can add one cubit to his stature? If you are not able to do the least, why are you anxious for the rest? Luke 12:22-26 NKJV

Start journaling your thoughts, fears, and prayers if you haven't already. It's essential to write down how you're feeling and document this experience because it helps you process your current state. It allows you to gain clarity about why you are in this place of suffering.

God's promises are contingent upon one thing: your love for His son, Jesus. Remember to ask in Jesus's name when you ask for His peace.

The Air That I Breathe

When you pray with love and gratitude, remember to pray in Jesus's name. When telling the enemy to leave your presence, say it in Jesus's name. There is no more powerful name underlined with grace than Jesus Christ. It's the greatest name ever given to the most incredible man who walked this earth. The impact it will have on your prayers and your life is tremendous.

Father God,

As the evening commences, I ask for peace and rest. Renew my spirit so the morning is energized and prepares me for another day walking with You.

I ask this in Jesus's name, amen.

Worship Song Suggestion:
I SPEAK JESUS
By, Here B Lions

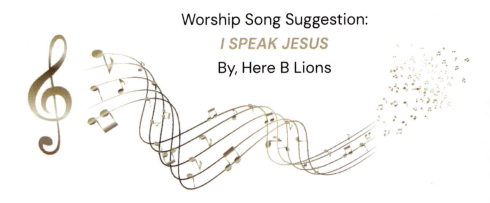

Jodi Howe

Take Aways:

Action Steps:

Day 7

I am an avid exerciser, not because I enjoy it, but because I want the results. I move my body as often as possible, whether walking or doing my favorite workout at the gym. Not only does it help my spirit, soul, and body, it encourages a discipline that we can equate to the results we get from reading the Bible.

His word helps to activate spiritual endorphins that positively effects our minds. Bible study builds a spiritual endurance during hard times, and offers an emotional assurance that God has everything under control.

Tip of the day: Get movin'!

For bodily exercise profits a little, but godliness is profitable for all things, having promise of the life that now is and of that which is to come. 1 Timothy 4:8 NKJV

Weather permitting, take a brisk walk and enjoy God's glorious gift of earth. If the weather doesn't help this, consider stretching or a moderate workout indoors. Try high impact or low impact workouts–even ten minutes at home from a healthy online activity will benefit you.

Honor the vessel God gave you by doing what you can to build its physical strength. Exercise pumps up your endorphins and improves your mood. Anxiety hates exercise, so let's tick it off today by doing something good for our bodies. You can do it!

We are not weak as anxiety sufferers, but it feels that way. It can be all-consuming. But take heart; God gets that. Isaiah reminds us that, through hope in God, our strength is renewed. We can rest assured that He is walking alongside us in our weakness and building us up with every breathe we offer to Him. Remember to surrender your day to Him. He loves hearing from us.

Dear Lord,

Today, as I put each step on the ground, remind me to look to You, the lifter of hope, spirit, and faith. I cannot approach this day alone, but I feel better already with You by my side. Thank You for Your grace and love for me.

In Jesus's glorious name, amen!

Take Aways:

Action Steps:

Night 7

One of my favorite parts of writing this book was finding worship songs to go with each day. I felt like a kid in a candy store. You should see my playlists.

Worship music feeds the spirit in the mind with good news and reminders of Jesus and His power and presence, especially during anxious moments. I would hear a worship song, and if I woke up fearful at night, I would repeatedly relay the music in my head. I promise you it works.

As a singer who serves on a worship team, I can attest to the power of music that has positive effects. This book speaks to how prayer is the bridge to panic and peace. And how music can bring about peace and, if chosen well, can bridge the gap between fear and peace. Worship music has been a life changer for me.

If you ever catch me on stage, you may find me jumping for joy.

 Tip of the night: Raise a hallelujah!

Let the word of Christ dwell in you richly in all wisdom, teaching and admonishing one another in psalms and hymns and spiritual songs, singing with grace in your hearts to the Lord. Colossians 3:16 NKJV

Nighttime can be unnerving. Trying to get a good night's sleep with overwhelming thoughts can be challenging. Listen to worship or calming music such as jazz, symphonic, etc. Hearing a worship song throughout the day or early night helps. By committing it to memory, when awakened with anxiety, you can run the lyrics through your head, which helps you feel at ease. Worship music is a form of prayer too!

The Air That I Breathe

Connecting to Jesus works wonders through Scripture, worship music, or simply talking to Him and sharing your fears by fervently asking for peace.

Prayer and petitioning your need for the Lord to "hold you tight throughout the night" is a great start.

Dear Jesus,

I'm letting fear and worry control my thoughts. This is the opposite of trusting You. Please come into my mind, control my thoughts, and lead me out of this darkness. Develop within me the confidence that a new day will dawn and new hope will rise.

In Your glorious name, amen.

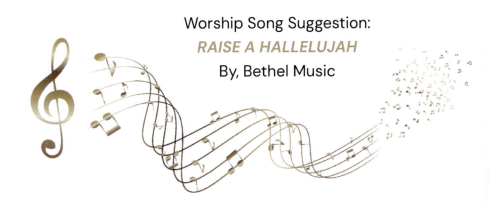

Worship Song Suggestion:
RAISE A HALLELUJAH
By, Bethel Music

Jodi Howe

Take Aways:

Action Steps:

7 Day Reflection

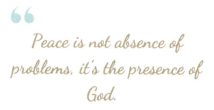
Peace is not absence of problems, it's the presence of God.

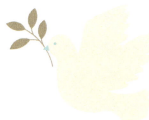

1. Have you tried a strategy that I recommended to ease anxiety? Yes or No?
   If so, what difference have you noticed this week?

   _____
   _____

   If not, review this past week and choose one that you can apply this week.

2. What was your favorite Bible verse this week? (Write it on some sticky notes and hang them everywhere or write it on a notecard and take it everywhere. Start memorizing it.)

   _____
   _____

3. What have you done to implement prayer at the start of your day? How has this helped you throughout the day?

   _____
   _____

If you haven't started the prayer process yet, no worries. You can start today.

Day 8

I was raised Italian; therefore, I was taught to eat a lot of food, but I still needed to learn to eat healthfully. My family and our world revolved around food. My Italian grandmothers used to have dinners daily, and I took advantage of that. Pasta, meatballs, cheese–the list was endless. The conversations around the tables were hysterical. But the food itself, as good as it tasted, wasn't always good for me.

Be mindful that you might need to pick and choose what you're eating while healing. But stay hopeful that one day, you will be able to indulge in a beautiful Italian dinner ... at least once in a while.

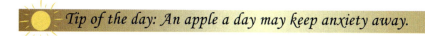
Tip of the day: An apple a day may keep anxiety away.

In the morning, LORD, you hear my voice; in the morning, I lay my requests before you and wait expectantly. Psalms 5:3 NIV

The food we eat has a significant impact on the level of anxiety we experience.

The following foods are high in nutrients we may be deficient in and can replace the components that encourage anxiety: apples, pumpkin seeds, specific herbal teas, avocados, almonds, lemons, salmon, turkey, oatmeal, bananas, and dark chocolate.

Consider avoiding certain foods that encourage weight gain and hyperactivity. These are typically high in sugar and make you feel crappy.

Dear Lord,

You've had my day planned from day one. I trust You with all my days. I ask that You reveal Yourself to me vividly, allowing me to see and hear You so I begin to know you better and better every day.
In Jesus's beautiful name, amen.

The Air That I Breathe

Take Aways:

Action Steps:

Night 8

This is a touchy subject, and I want to be clear that many things revolve around alcohol and alcoholism. I'm not about lecturing. But I am about to warn you that during your process of healing, alcohol will not be your friend. Take this from someone who used it to medicate, almost to the point of being addicted.

I am grateful I didn't have to learn the hard way, and I pray you do not either. And even if you're reading this right now and suffer from alcoholism, remember that today is a new day, and healing is possible.

For now, it's best to avoid consuming alcohol.

Tip of the night: Consume the Holy Spirit.

Or do you not know that your body is the temple of the Holy Spirit who is in you, whom you have from God, and you are not your own? For you were bought at a price; therefore glorify God in your body and in your spirit, which are God's. 1 Corinthians 6:19-20 NKJV

Alcohol is both a sedative and a depressant that affects the central nervous system. Alcohol changes levels of serotonin and other neurotransmitters in the brain. This can make your anxiety worse. Although in the short term, it promotes the feeling of "taking the edge off" and makes you feel less anxious, in the long term, you may begin to feel even more nervous after the alcohol wears off.

As you work to understand anxiety and how it affects your livelihood, there are many triggers and things you should avoid as you get a grasp on this illness. Many foods and alcohol can encourage more anxiety, and that's exactly what we're trying to avoid. Medical professionals strongly suggest that as you try to get a grip on living with less stress,

The Air That I Breathe

avoid alcohol and foods high in salts, sugars, processed ingredients, and unhealthy fats.

Father God,

Anxiety is a form of suffering I don't want to have in my life. However, I know I can't completely control the diminishing of this disease by myself. I need Your grace and internal peace to know I will have my life back again. A life filled with joy and grace is part of Your many promises.

It's in your Son's beautiful name I pray this to you. amen.

Worship Song Suggestion:
HEALING BEGINS
By, Tenth Avenue North

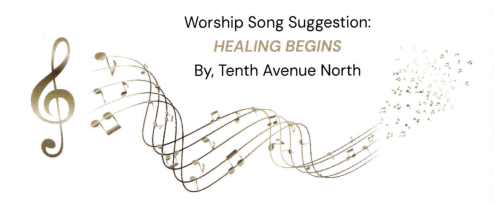

Jodi Howe

Take Aways:

Action Steps:

Day 9

Do you remember the saying, "The mind is a powerful thing to waste?" It's so true. What we feed our minds can be damaging. I had to be aware of what I watched on television in order to protect my mind and all that flowed through it. When I didn't, negativity overpowered me, and I became fearful, anxious, and doubted I would ever find peace.

I had to be careful about the music I listened to and the social media I participated in. I also had to be mindful of whom I spent time with, which included family members and friends. My circle decreased until I was well on my way to healing. Temporarily, that is. I am back to being the cute social butterfly God created me to be.

 Tip of the day: Mind over matter.

For "who has known the mind of the Lord that he may instruct Him?" But we have the mind of Christ. 1 Corinthians 2:16 NKJV

Do your best to stay positive and peaceful. Avoid negativity, anger, frustration, and people that cause it. This includes social media. It has pros and cons. But the cons are powerful. They can exasperate anxiety.

This may be easier said than done, but negativity makes anxiety thrive. It's not our intention to be in unhealthy relationships or have family members who are challenging to deal with; this may be unavoidable.

However, as you begin healing your own heart and gripping your anxiety disorder, you may have to limit the amount of time shared around negative people and social media, because others' circumstances often become yours. Putting your mental health first can be the start of allowing you to feel stronger and better equipped to handle negativity and toxicity. Your intent is good because you are

trying to heal from your anxiety. And it's okay to set boundaries so you can recover.

Father God,

There are negative people and circumstances in this free world, and sometimes it encourages my anxiety. I ask that You bring peace to my heart and personal space so I can heal and grow closer to you.

In Jesus's beautiful name, amen.

Take Aways:

Action Steps:

Night 9

*L*earning that my life is not about me has been a tough spiritual muscle to flex. Yet when I realized that God is in control and I could lean on Him through everything, and I mean *everything*, a massive weight off of my anxious shoulders dissipated.

When I learned that peace is not the absence of problems, it's the presence of God, I saw that the more I worried, the more I avoided God. Living for the world is unsustainable because the world is filled with broken sinners like me. The world is a problem creator. It can't help me. But God can. He is the ultimate redeemer.

Tip of the night: He is God; you are not!

Therefore we do not lose heart. Even though our outward man is perishing, yet the inward man is being renewed day by day. For our light affliction, which is but for a moment, is working for us a far more exceeding and eternal weight of glory, while we do not look at the things which are seen, but at the things which are not seen. For the things which are seen are temporary, but the things which are not seen are eternal. 2 Corinthians 4:16–18 NKJV

Do your best to avoid going to bed with the world's weight on your shoulders. If you had a difficult day that may have included arguments, conflict, or frustrating circumstances, tomorrow is a new day and new hope. Keep your eyes on Jesus, and ask Him to bring in His promised peace.

Problems are a part of life and, in some instances, unavoidable. But as you build a stronger relationship with Jesus Christ, you will see that troubles can be momentary, and the mental load will lighten because your trust in Him can bring miraculous peace even through

The Air That I Breathe

brutal storms. You will start to see that some problems in your life manifested because you took them on unnecessarily, but as you give your concerns to the Lord, you'll be amazed at how they get rectified. In His way, with His will, and in His time. Just stay loyal and trusting, and He will do the same threefold.

Father God,

Problems surround me daily, and I know they're a part of life, but I want to learn to experience a presence in this world to include joy and peace that only You can provide. Life is not without conflict, but You overcame the world so that I can overcome my trials with You by my side.

In Jesus's name, amen!

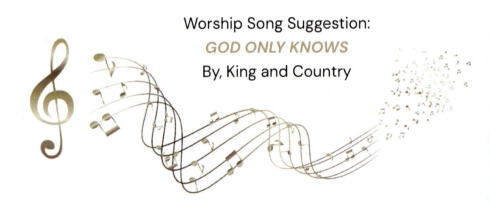

Worship Song Suggestion:
GOD ONLY KNOWS
By, King and Country

Jodi Howe

Take Aways:

Action Steps:

Day 10

I know this may sound redundant to anxiety, but stay busy within reason. If God is telling you to be still, heed that voice. Remember, God rested on the seventh day and made a rest day for us too.

On working days, when you have anxious moments, don't stay prisoner to those thoughts. Consider going for a walk, cleaning, or organizing. When I felt out of control, I looked for productive tasks. As a stay-at-home mom, there was always something to do. And for the short-term, it worked.

My long-term solution is always prayer and the Word of God.

Tip of the day: Rely while you occupy.

In the morning sow your seed, And in the evening do not withhold your hand; For you do not know which will prosper, Either this or that, Or whether both alike will be good. Ecclesiastes 11:6 NKJV

If you work at home, keep yourself busy with cleaning, organizing, walking the dog, cooking, crafts, and whatever keeps your mind off anxiety.

If you work out of the home and sit at a desk all day or even drive a lot, give yourself a break throughout the day. Go outside for fresh air or window shop during a work break.

Try to keep your mind and body busy with productive thoughts. Remember, worrying is not practical.

As sufferers of anxiety, we simply long for peace. Peace of mind, heart, soul, thoughts, actions, reactions—you name it, we yearn for it. Jesus

Jodi Howe

left us the gift of peace, and like all gifts, we must remember to be gracious and accept it with love and trust.

Father God,

As I walk into this day, which could most definitely include trouble and problems, I ask that You immediately bring me to a place of peace and remind me that I need to stand firm, that Your gift of peace is solid, and that I am worthy of it, always.

In His precious name, amen!

The Air That I Breathe

Take Aways:

Action Steps:

Jodi Howe

Night 10

When I was a teenager, I was not in good shape, but in order for me to get a spot on my high school's dance team, I had to get fit. The audition process consisted of working out in the hot summer heat with the marching band. That is where I discovered the benefits of drinking lots of water.

I consume water in abundance to this day, enjoying hydration's incredible benefits for the spirit, soul, and body. My water bottle collection is a bit much, but my water intake is always maintained. Fun fact: water is also great for your complexion, hair, and nails.

Tip of the night: *Heaven's hydration.*

O God, You are my God; Early will I seek You; My soul thirsts for You; My flesh longs for You in a dry and thirsty land Where there is no water. Psalm 63:1 NKJV

Avoid eating heavy foods or eating late at night. Fatty food before you go to bed can cause a slew of problems and can interrupt your much-needed, peaceful sleep. Remember to drink water (recommended, 6-8 glasses) throughout the day. Hydration is essential and has a refreshing effect when anxious.

Not only do you have to keep your body well fueled and hydrated, but it's also essential to keep your mind hydrated with the Word of God, especially at night when anxiety can peak and rear its ugly head.

If you haven't had the chance to read the Bible or even open one, please do.

The Gospels are stories of Jesus. What a great place to start. They are in the New Testament with four interpretations from Matthew, Mark, Luke, and John.

The Air That I Breathe

Read the apostle Paul's books, which are profound missions: discerning and strengthening one's spirit. Teaching us to get to the heart of the matter.

In the Old Testament, David's writings in Psalms are compelling, as he, too, suffered from much, but because his heart was for God, he was given incredible mercy and grace.

Don't forget the book of Job. Job's obedience and devotion towards God during his most profound sorrow provided a pathway to God's tender mercy and renewal of life.

And so on!

The Bible is God's love story to us. Fall in love with Jesus tonight.

Dear God,

Your Bible is a love story to us. It's filled with so much that we can benefit from daily. Please lead me to Your Word and remind me that your wisdom can become mine. Thank You for the Bible, this day, and the daily bread You provided among the many gifts You blessed me with.

In His precious name, amen!

Worship Song Suggestion:
WORD OF GOD SPEAK
By, Mercy Me

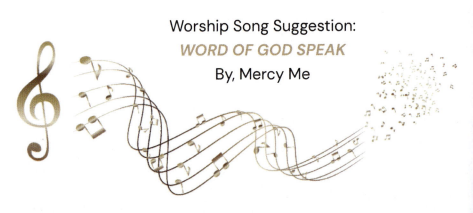

Jodi Howe

Take Aways:

Action Steps:

Day 11

The stigma around anxiety and mental illness is high but not as high as in years past. As you know, my testimony shows how my fear was instigated because of the stigma. But our human condition has ailments. That's a part of our broken world.

The sooner I accepted that anxiety was my reality but not my identity, the sooner I lived peacefully. I now see why anxiety escalated in my life. It was so God could use it for my growth and to aid in helping others grow in Him.

Tip of the Day: Acceptance is not defeat when you understand anxiety's relevance as a part of life.

He who walks with wise men will be wise, But the companion of fools will be destroyed. Proverbs 13:20 NKJV

Acceptance is crucial to the realization that you may have a mental illness.

Yet you're not alone in the suffering, and it is essential to remember that the world suffers from hundreds of illnesses every day. Because those illnesses are part of our reality, the stigma needs to be erased.

Mental illness is like any other disease, such as cancer, heart disease, or diabetes. No one has asked to suffer from anxiety; it's disheartening, but take heart; it is manageable.

There are excellent resources, doctors, therapies, medicines, support groups, and so much to help you learn to live with anxiety and not let it debilitate your days and livelihood.

And the most beautiful thought you should always take away from your suffering is that the Lord loves you and doesn't want to see you suffer.

Jodi Howe

Dear Lord Jesus,

Please walk with me as I have moments of disappointment and sadness. As I realize I am not perfect, I know You are. You came to save me from sin and give us the promise of eternal life, and I need You more than ever in my life right now. I wish I didn't have to deal with anxiety, but I know You came to the cross to heal me. The cross represents how Your beautiful sacrifice allows me to live abundantly. You overcame the world; I'm confident that I can overcome anxiety. And with that, I want to thank You for the cross.

In Your son's name, amen.

The Air That I Breathe

Take Aways:

Action Steps:

Night 11

"Let go and let God" is a stable talking point in Christian dialogue, yet we still fight it. I get it. I am a work in progress since I, too, struggle with handing it all over to God.

Consider the practice of intentionally surrendering to God. It helps to quiet racing minds and keeps us from ruminating on the day's problems.

Let's continue to try to do that together.

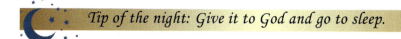

Tip of the night: Give it to God and go to sleep.

The LORD replied, "My Presence will go with you, and I will give you rest." Exodus 33:14 NIV

Before you go to bed, give your sleep to Jesus. Tell Him you're worried about fear creeping into the night and that you pray for a peaceful sleep. Even if you wake up in the middle of the night, know you can turn your mind to Him. His grace will bestow that peace He repeatedly promises in Scripture.

My sleep has always been essential to me; for the most part, I've been an excellent sleeper. However, anxiety can affect your sleep. In addition to many of the tips in this book, I found that if you stay focused on Jesus, whether in prayer, worship, or reading Scripture, He will give you that sweet sleep you so desperately desire.

Dear God,

On the seventh day, You rested. And our bodies need it daily. My fear is overwhelming and is keeping me awake. I ask that You work within my mind to bring me to a place of peace so I can slumber away and praise You the next day. In Jesus's name, amen.

The Air That I Breathe

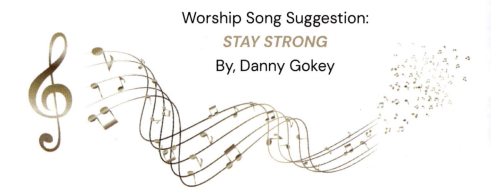

Worship Song Suggestion:
STAY STRONG
By, Danny Gokey

Jodi Howe

Take Aways:

Action Steps:

The Air That I Breathe

Day 12

Anxiety didn't care that I was married, had a lovely home, an established life, or was healthy. It reared its ugly head and will do so to anyone, anywhere, in any way it wants to.

Male, female, young, old, any race, any ethnicity, all of us can be culprits to anxiety. I'm learning that this does not make you weak but strong when you deal with it.

 Tip of the day: Anxiety does not discriminate.

He gives the power to the weak, And to those who have no might He increases strength. Even the youths shall faint and be weary, And the young men shall utterly fall, But those who wait on the LORD shall renew their strength; They shall mount up with wings like eagles, They shall run and not be weary, They shall walk and not faint. Isaiah 40:29–31 NKJV

Hormones, negative thoughts, specific events, and various things tremendously affect anxiety for both men and women. Understand the signs and take control of your symptoms before you allow your mind to crash into a severe panic attack.

Anxiety is not necessarily out of the blue. Here are some potential triggers:

- Unfortunate events or milestones
- Hormones
- Health crisis
- News
- Negative thoughts
- People (even family and friends)
- Poor diet
- PTSD

Know that there are tremendous factors that intensify anxiety. When you are anxious, see if the above triggers it, and then do your best to use the strategies I talk about in this book to heal your body.

You are strong and must be reminded that Christ is the Prince of Peace, and no giant can defeat us when we are under His power.

Go to the Bible. Open it up to 1 Samuel, Chapter 17. Read it. It's the story of David and Goliath. See how God can use anyone to defeat anything that seems giant in our lives.

Dear Lord,

Many factors encourage anxiety, and I need to be aware of them. Through prayer, I need to draw You closer. Use the wisdom You provide to combat my anxiety. I pray for that wisdom from You.

In Jesus's name, amen.

The Air That I Breathe

Take Aways:

Action Steps:

Night 12

The *wise mind* became a saving grace for panic attacks. I heard it on a podcast years ago, and wow, it works. The wise mind overrides the fearful and anxious thoughts that are counterproductive. I learned to stop listening to my emotional mind, which was bullying me. Using common sense, I could control and defeat nonsensical thinking.

> *Tip of the night: Use your "wise mind" to rid your crazy thoughts.*

Whenever I am afraid, I will trust in you. In God (I will praise His word), In God I have put my trust. Psalm 56:3-4 NKJV

If you feel anxiety and panic coming on, before you hit the fight or flight button, use your wise mind to remind you it's just anxiety, and you can overcome it.

I learned about the **Wise Mind** and found it a game changer when anxiety and panic overpower me with **Crazy Thoughts**. Slowly but surely, you will begin to know what those are:

- Racing thoughts
- Obsessive-compulsive disorder
- Constant worrying
- Numbing with drugs and alcohol
- Safety rituals or superstitions
- Over preparing
- Hypochondria
- Seeking out Dr. Google for remedies

And so much more. As mentioned, meditation is key to anxiety, and by taking those "crazy thoughts" out of your mind and replacing them with common sense, you find freedom from anxiety.

The Air That I Breathe

Here is a great meditation when you are feeling anxiety and panic.

- Take your fist and place it on your stomach right above your hips and under your ribs.
- Breathe in for five seconds through your nose.
- Breathe out for five seconds out through your mouth.

This helps to remind yourself that your "wise mind" is taking control of your "crazy thoughts," and you begin to believe that this exercise will bring you to a place of relaxation and peace.

Sometimes, shifting the focus of your mind onto another area helps to reiterate that you have this control and can avoid your thoughts getting the best of you.

Dear Lord,

Our minds are powerful instruments made to bring us thoughtfully through life. I ask that You allow my "wise mind" to step in when my "crazy thoughts" try to get the best of me. It seems the enemy is trying to hurt me, yet only You can make him leave my mind in the name of Jesus Christ! I'm so grateful for You and Your healing.

In Jesus's name, amen.

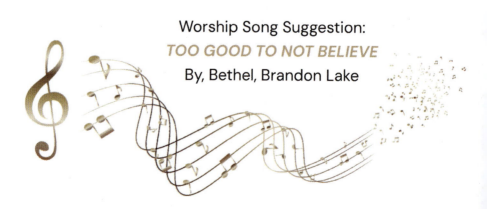

Worship Song Suggestion:
TOO GOOD TO NOT BELIEVE
By, Bethel, Brandon Lake

Jodi Howe

Take Aways:

Action Steps:

Day 13

*M*y prayer is to help you overcome anxiety with God's power. I also pray you begin a deeper relationship with Him.

I am endlessly in love with the Lord Jesus Christ. In addition to His healing, Jesus has become my foundation through trials and tribulations. His tests, provisions, and discernment have brought me to a deeper level of hope and gratitude than ever before.

I see His beauty more clearly. When I walk by the ocean, I feel Him walking with me. When I see a baby, I see His miracles. When the seasons change, I am amazed at how God's canvas becomes a new work of art.

I seek His wisdom more earnestly. I appreciate His gifts and blessings. They are all around us. We just have to open our spiritual eyes to see them.

Tip of the day: April showers bring May flowers.

> Then He arose and rebuked the wind, and said to the sea, "Peace, be still!" And the wind ceased and there was a great calm. Mark 4:39 NKJV

Enjoy God's beauty. Take a walk in a garden, or search a floral site online. See the fantastic nature the Lord gifts us with every day. Even after a torrential rain or windy storm, nature bounces right back. So can you!

You will encounter many storms throughout your life, and no doubt the "mental storms" can take a considerable toll, causing anxiety to heighten during times of stress, pain, loss, and hurt.

Remember to praise God through your storms, as He is doing tremendous work in you. If you stay focused on Him, you will grow and prosper in spirit, life, relationships, and trials. I am a testimony to that.

Jodi Howe

Father God,

I am scared and anxious that this storm will never pass. Please show up in ways to assure me that You have calmed the angry seas. In faith, You can ease my anxious mind.

In Your son's name, I pray, amen.

The Air That I Breathe

Take Aways:

Action Steps:

Night 13

The power of love in my life assures me there is a God. God is love, and He provides that through relationships. Nothing compares to His love, yet some beautiful souls work hard to replicate it. And it's a beautiful thing I see in my children, parents, and friends. With Jesus, I now walk with love.

> *Tip of the night: Love can move mountains.*

Love suffers long and is kind; love does not envy; love does not parade itself, is not puffed up; does not behave rudely, does not seek its own, is not provoked, thinks no evil; does not rejoice in iniquity, but rejoices in the truth; bears all things, believes all things, hopes all things, endures all things. 1 Corinthians 13:4–7 NKJV

I encourage focusing on love to end your evening. If you are married, snuggle your spouse. Hug and love your children. Adore those pets of yours. If you are alone, call a loved one and share a fun story. Don't get caught up in life's loneliness. Jesus is a comforter. Jesus is love.

Love is a powerful tool that can break the chains of many bonds we suffer from. Expressing love to your spouse, mate, children, pets, family, and friends holds no boundaries. It's not projected in a selfish nature. Love can calm the senses and raise your mood tremendously. End your evenings with love on your mind.

Dear Lord,

I love you! I know You loved me and the whole world so much; You sacrificed Your Son, and He suffered to give me this life. That love never dies. I want to spend every day offering love to all who enter my pathway. Please infuse me with that ability always.
In Jesus's name, amen!

The Air That I Breathe

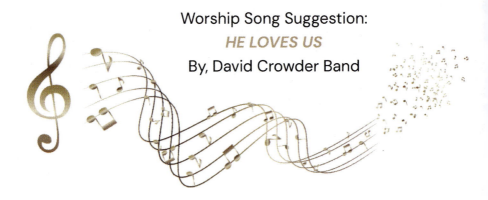

Worship Song Suggestion:
HE LOVES US
By, David Crowder Band

P.S. I cry every time I listen to this song.

Take Aways:

Action Steps:

The Air That I Breathe

Day 14

*H*ere's that breathing tip again. But it's critical for anxiety, singing, childbirth, and exercise ... need I go on? Although I am afraid to scuba dive (still considering snorkeling), I trust I am a good breather because I have intentionally strengthened this muscle whenever I need it. So please do yourself a favor: breathe better.

Tip of the day: Here is a breathe of fresh air.

As long as my breath is in me, and the breathe of God in my nostrils, My lips will not speak wickedness, Nor my tongue utter deceit. Job 27:3-4 NKJV

Become a *"nose breather."* Breathing through your nose is more effective than mouth breathing. This can be practiced in meditation. Balancing the oxygen and carbon dioxide ratio helps to avoid hyperventilation.

Yes, we do breathe incorrectly. As a singer, I know this very well. Poor breathing can encourage anxiety. If you start feeling anxious, focus on breathing by breathing in through your nose and out through your mouth. It can help avoid your fear factor, causing you to hyperventilate into full-fledged panic attacks.

Consider doing this amid a beautiful aromatherapy scent. I always encourage lavender.

Father God,

You created me uniquely and beautifully, yet the human body complex. Please keep me focused on good breathing practices so I can breathe in your grace daily and exhale your peace.
In Jesus's Name, amen.

Take Aways:

Action Steps:

Night 14

"What? I am not the only one suffering from anxiety?"

No, you are not. Reality checks are essential.

The best form of gratitude in healing is to hope for others' success. I have prayed over this book. I have prayed that it helps you to heal. And I will continue to do so. How about joining me in prayers for others?

> *Tip of the night: Be generous and pray for others tonight!*

And you, child, will be called the prophet of the Highest; For you will go before the face of the Lord to prepare His ways, To give knowledge of salvation to His people By the remission of their sins, Through the tender mercy of our God, With which the Dayspring from on high has visited us; To give light to those who sit in darkness and the shadow of death, To guide our feet into the way of peace." Luke 1:76-79 NKJV

Take a moment tonight to pray for those suffering from anxiety. Whether you know them or not, ask God to give them strength and peace in their struggles.

And if you know someone who suffers from anxiety, share some hope today.

If you have felt inspiration from this book within the last few weeks, please share what you have learned with others. It is my prayer and hope that we rely on the hope of God and His possibilities of healing through anxiety in our communities.

God tells us we are to give light to those who sit in darkness and feel the shadows of death surrounding them. Be that light.

Jodi Howe

Dear Lord,

I am not the only one suffering from this disease. I ask that You lay your strong hand on all those suffering from anxiety so that they are brought peace and relief. Bring them healing through fellowship, church, reading, medicine, or whatever your will is to show them the light in their current darkness. And if I can aid as a human vessel, please guide and direct my next steps. You are so good.

In Jesus's name, amen!

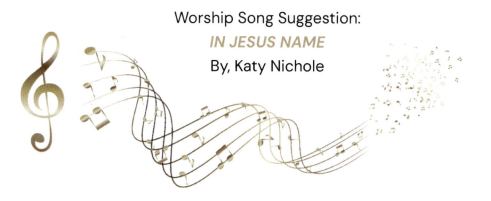

Worship Song Suggestion:
IN JESUS NAME
By, Katy Nichole

Take Aways:

Action Steps:

14 Day Reflection

> *Prayer is the bridge between panic and peace.*

1. How are you changing your diet and what you expose yourself to?
   _____
   _____

   Have you noticed a difference in how you are feeling?
   _____
   _____

   If you haven't started yet, consider starting this week.

2. What have you done to feed your mind with good, positive, and inspiring things?
   _____
   _____

   Write down books you've found and new podcasts you are listening to.
   _____
   _____

3. Has your trust in God helped you with anxious moments lately?
   _____
   _____

Trust that everything will work out and have faith that God is guiding you.

Jodi Howe

Day 15

Disorganization, chaos, and poor planning love hanging out with anxiety. I used to become overwhelmed by those things, but I now get ahead by planning my life better. Of course, we will make plans, but the Lord will direct our steps. Preparing my day is my responsibility and directing my steps, is God's. Preparation is key to preventing unnecessary anxiety throughout the day.

I am an over packer, a notetaker, and a go with "God's flow" kind of girl. What a fun combination He has created in me. You are also fearfully and wonderfully made and your combination is perfect for you.

Tip of the day: Day planner.

Commit your works to the LORD, And your thoughts will be established. Proverbs 16:3 NKJV

Prepare your day as it *should* look, not how you fear it *will* look.

Write a list of positive expectations to avoid focusing on anxiety. If you love planners or technical lists, or even sticky notes, start your day with a plan to stay positive and productive.

Include being grateful for the good times with your best efforts to enjoy the day's blessings. Do all this by writing a list of positive expectations.

Father God,

I may wake up in fear, but if I focus on You, there will be tremendous blessings throughout the day, to which my anxiety will try to close my eyes. Please open my eyes to see Your beauty in every walk I take today. Please discern my steps.
It's in His name I pray this, amen.

Take Aways:

Action Steps:

Night 15

I cherish my sleep if you haven't figured it out by now.

I discovered natural plants that help aid our sleep and have to share them with you. I've always known about lavender, but the others were also cool to discover.

Hey, it can't hurt!

 Tip of the night: Plant yourself to sleep!

Now may the Lord of peace Himself give you peace always and in every way. The Lord be with you all. 2 Thessalonians 3:16 NKJV

Wow, who knew even a plant could give us peace? Never underestimate the power of nature in the botanical world.

Below is a list of plants proven to produce additional "positive energy oxygen" while you sleep.

- Aloe Vera: Emits oxygen at night, improves sleep quality and insomnia.
- Lavender Plant: Helps induce sleep and reduce anxiety, slows down heart rate.
- Jasmine Plant: Improves quality of sleep, increases productivity and alertness, and reduces anxiety.
- English Ivy: Reduces air molds, benefits people with asthma and breathing problems.
- Snake Plant: Emits oxygen, takes away carbon dioxide from the air, and filters nasty toxins.

The Air That I Breathe

Dear Father,

Thank You for Your earthly gifts that have calming results. Your earth supplies so much healing, and I am so grateful You care so much about me that You had these remedies planned from the start.

In Your Son's name, amen.

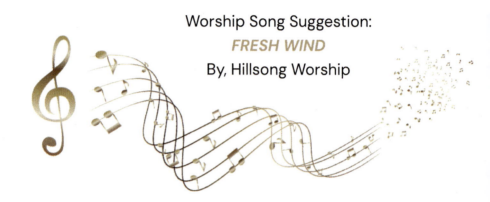

Worship Song Suggestion:
FRESH WIND
By, Hillsong Worship

Jodi Howe

Take Aways:

_____
_____
_____
_____
_____
_____
_____

Action Steps:

_____
_____
_____
_____
_____
_____
_____

The Air That I Breathe

Day 16

Since I am sharing so much, I will confess this. I am a neat freak. I am imperfect, but I work towards tidiness, organization, and avoiding clutter. It takes effort, but it limits so much anxiety. Things have a place and should be put back in those places. All rooms in my home (except in my teenage daughter's room, sigh, this is where I would insert the angry emoji) are neat and in order. I don't leave dishes hanging around. Clothes are not on the floor. My home stays neat.

Therefore, my head stays neat as well.

I am still working on my daughter.

Tip of the day: Tidy up your mind.

Let all things be done decently and in order. 1 Corinthians 14:40 NKJV

One of the best ways I've found to clear my mind is to clear the area around me.

The clutter of our surroundings and belongings becomes the clutter in our minds. Start decluttering by going through your belongings and saying, "Is this important, or is it simply taking up space I don't have?" Or ask yourself, When was the last time I used this? Can this benefit someone else?"

Categorizing items in closets and cabinets helps eliminate products you are no longer using. Make piles of clothes and other things to donate and feel great about knowing that what you consider junk could make someone else's day by becoming their new treasure.

Father God, I pray the clutter in my mind can be reduced as I declutter my surroundings. Please motivate me to reorganize my home, mind, body, and spirit.

In Jesus's name, amen.

Take Aways:

Action Steps:

Night 16

The world confuses feelings for facts. Take, for example these secular sayings: "trust your gut, seek happiness first, and you've got this." These particular worldly affirmations have challenged me throughout life.

Truth bomb here: We should not trust our feelings!

I experience such freedom because I have shifted this perspective. Feelings are data. The Holy Spirit is the processor. Jesus has the answers. It's that simple.

 Tip of the night: Filter your feelings.

That He would grant you, according to the riches of His glory, to be strengthened with might through His Spirit in the inner man, that Christ may dwell in your hearts through faith; that you, being rooted and grounded in love, may be able to comprehend with all the saints what is the width and length and depth and height—to know the love of Christ which passes knowledge; that you may be filled with all of the fullness of God. Ephesians 3:16-19 NKJV

Feelings aren't always factual and may not steer you in the right direction. Feelings should be used as data to be broken down and better discerned when guided by wisdom and common sense.

Our anxious minds can convince us we are shameful, guilt-ridden, lowly, fearful people. And although our feelings are our feelings, they may not be helpful towards productive healing.

Is the glass half full or half empty? This is a choice we make every day. Negative thoughts cause negative feelings, but positive thoughts can create calmness and joy.

Unconsciously, we think negatively and react more with our feelings and less with our wise minds. As you go into a negative thought process, stop yourself and say, "Is this a productive way to think?" Most likely it's not. However, you can have a peaceful mind. That's a fact.

Filter your feelings through God in prayer. Ask Him if this thought or feeling is coming from Him.

Father God,

Please encourage my mind to stay focused on You, as that will help to keep my mind calm, peaceful, and positive. You are the most favorable light in this world and the best part of our days and nights.

In Your Son's name, amen.

Worship Song Suggestion:
BUILD MY LIFE
By, Housefires

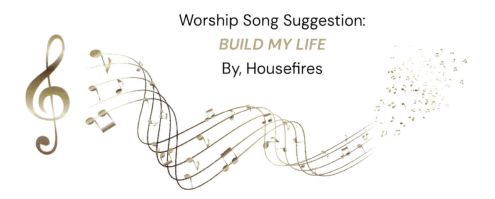

Take Aways:

Action Steps:

Jodi Howe

Day 17

Anxiety has the potential to debilitate us. I was immobilized by travel. I was terrified to fly, and it kept me close to home. I avoided events with people I desperately wanted to see and trips I wanted to take because I was afraid to fly. I missed adventure. I missed God's canvas.

Since God has healed my anxiety, He has reintroduced me to His world, and I have begun to yearn for more exploration. I even bought a new set of luggage that I'm excited to use.

 Tip of the day: Take a day trip.

The Lord is my shepherd; I shall not want. He makes me to lie down in green pastures; He leads me beside the still waters. He restores my soul; He leads me in the paths of righteousness For His name's sake. Psalms 23:1-3 NKJV

Our world is filled with so much beauty. There are beautiful places to visit within hours of your home. Beaches, lakes, waterfalls, mountains. Exciting and charming destinations await you. I know I sound like a timeshare here, but it's a newfound excitement the Lord has shown me.

I encourage you to "treat yourself" as a remedy to anxiety. Believe that a change of scenery may give you time to clear your mind so you can be in the presence of Christ.

The Air That I Breathe

Dear Father,

When I feel let down and anxious, I take my spirit to a place of peace and beauty. You have blessed us with so many beautiful places on this earth. Direct me to that blessing today.

In Jesus's name, amen.

Take Aways:

Action Steps:

Night 17

I know, I know, I talk too much about sleep. We don't value it enough, and lack of sleep can lead to anxiety. My bedroom is a sanctuary. My sanctuary. When I sleep better, I pray and read His Word better. I am better to my people. I am better for the world. So, sweet dreams.

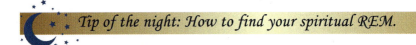

Tip of the night: How to find your spiritual REM.

When you lie down, you will not be afraid; Yes, you will lie down and your sleep will be sweet. Proverbs 3:24 NKJV

Get to sleep and stay there! (For at least 7 hours.)

1. **Stick to a sleep schedule with the same bedtime and wake-up time, even on the weekends.** This helps to regulate your body's clock and can help you fall asleep and stay asleep for the night.
2. **Practice a relaxing bedtime ritual.** A relaxing routine right before bedtime, away from bright lights, helps separate your sleep time from activities that can cause excitement, stress, or anxiety. All of these things make it more difficult to fall asleep, get sound and deep sleep, or remain asleep.
3. **Avoid naps if you have trouble sleeping.** I am a fan of power naps, but if you can't fall asleep at bedtime, eliminating even short catnaps may help.
4. **Exercise daily.** Vigorous exercise is best, but light exercise is better than no activity. It's fine at any time of day, but not at the expense of your sleep.
5. **Sleep on a comfortable mattress and pillows.** Make sure your bed is comfortable and supportive. For most good quality mattresses, the one you have used for years may have exceeded its life

expectancy—about nine or ten years. Have comfortable pillows and make the room attractive and inviting for sleep.

6. **Try sleep blankets.** Sleep blankets promote deep touch pressure, or DTP, by applying gentle, distributed pressure on the body, which has been shown to increase serotonin. Serotonin, the chemical in the body that helps regulate mood and has a calming effect, benefits people with anxiety.

Dear God,

Now I lay me down to sleep, I pray to You, my soul to keep. May the angels watch me through the night until I wake till morning light.

In Jesus's precious name, amen.

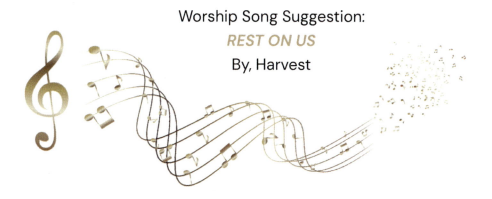

Worship Song Suggestion:
REST ON US
By, Harvest

Take Aways:

Action Steps:

Day 18

My college graduation is where my anxiety began. And then it was a move to the west coast. And then it was a milestone birthday. Do you see the trajectory? All milestones.

I could have gotten ahead if I had known then what I know now. But it's all good now that God has equipped me to understand Him better. And after you read this book, you will know better too.

 Tip of the day: Milestones are life markers, not fear factors.

And we know that all things work together for good to those who love God, to those who are called according to His purpose. For whom He foreknew, He also predestined to be conformed to the image of His Son, that He might be the first born among many brethren. Moreover whom He predestined, these He also called; whom He called, these He also justified; and whom He justified, these He also glorified. Romans 8:28-30 NKJV

A high school or college graduation, a plan for marriage, a new job or career change, postpartum depression, a milestone birthday (21, 30, 40, 50 +), and so many other turning points—anxiety gets its fill in our lives through life markers.

My testimony began with a life marker that became a fear-monger and incrementally interfered with my life's plans.

Please don't allow it to overpower your time of change and celebration. Remind yourself you will not be ruled by anxiety, as God (and He alone) wants us to live an abundant life filled with joy. Celebrate and thank God for your blessings and those beautiful milestones that remind us of the glories He gives us on earth.

The Air That I Breathe

Aging brings about more wisdom, which is priceless. Yet, I will still support anti-aging facial products.

Dear Father,

As this current chapter ends, I await for what's in store for my new chapter, as I trust You will be by my side. Please continue to shed hope and love as fuel for my glorious days on earth. With much gratitude for all Your blessings,

In Jesus's name, amen.

Take Aways:

Action Steps:

Night 18

*T*echnology is a double-edged sword. You may be reading this on a device.

I grew up in the not-so-techno world. But it was evolving. Faster than ever. I can see the good in it, but also the bad. I am writing a book on it. I am also checking texts and social media here or there for some emotional catch-up.

To be clear, our minds work better without technology because it distracts us. You get the picture.

 Tip of the night: Technically speaking ...

And do not be conformed to this world, but be transformed by the renewing of your mind, that you may prove what is that good and acceptable and perfect will of God. Romans 12:2 NKJV

Before you go to bed, turn electronic devices off.

iPhones, iPads, laptops, and TVs are the way of the world, yet they are a double-edged sword.

This subject is probably a book on its own. We do hold the world in our pockets through a smart device. Is it making us more intelligent, though? Or helping our mental health?

Sitting in bed with a tablet or screen works against us when we're trying to fall asleep.

Research has shown that the lights on most electronic screens have the most potential to influence and delay the body's natural circadian rhythms, making it harder to fall asleep. Keep your TVs out of your bedroom and unplug your devices. Keep good books on the nightstand.

Because, like me, we all know our phones will be waiting for us bright and early in the morning.

Dear Father,

Our modern world makes it hard not to want to constantly be "in the know" or encourage our addictions to social media. Please give me discernment to honor my sleep time with quiet time, gearing my focus on You through prayer and meditation.

In Your Son's name, amen.

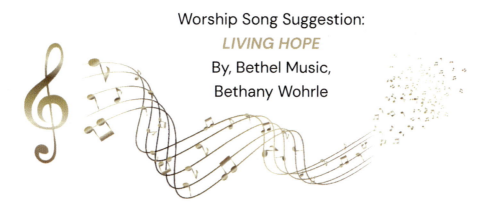

Worship Song Suggestion:
LIVING HOPE
By, Bethel Music,
Bethany Wohrle

Take Aways:

Action Steps:

Day 19

I have been walking with Christ for twelve years now. But it wasn't until the great pandemic of our generation that I learned about the fullness of the power of the Holy Spirit. My spiritual growth soared.

A spiritual maturity evolved when I learned that the Holy Spirit is the faithful intercessor, communicator, and connector to God in heaven.

I experienced a revival in my ministry.

 Tip of the day: Flex on the power of the Holy Spirit.

But the Helper, the Holy Spirit, whom the Father will send in My name, He will teach you all things, and bring to your remembrance all things that I said to you. John 14:26 NKJV

We all have idiosyncrasies. Mine are:

- I am not a morning person.
- I was a white knuckle flyer.
- I feared death.

It's incredible to think I could ever function, right? I function because of the skills I developed from understanding and accepting anxiety as my personal health concern. In addition, I discovered that I needed to utilize the Holy Spirit. The gift sent to me from God, through Jesus Christ. I can flex on this powerful Spirit and seek Him out in a time of need—the transmitter to the Holy God of the universe Himself. This shift in perspective became a game changer.

When we invite him into our hearts, He lives inside of us twenty-four seven. He gives us power. The Holy Trinity has three ways to hear, walk, and talk with God. Utilizing the Holy Spirit is critical while we navigate this tricky world.

I am a new creation in God. In addition to His wisdom, discernment, and direction, He gave me a brain that functions. Therefore, I can act accordingly. I'm perfectly capable of applying practical measures to calm those fears.

So, I have to be attentive to the following.

I need to ease my way into the day so I don't develop anxiety. This means waking up earlier than necessary to allow me that much-needed time to "wake up" naturally. Coffee included.

I have had a severe fear of flying. I know *all* the facts and statistics; I don't enjoy the ride. I used to need medication to fly. No longer. However, I need mental preparation, meditation, music, and a window seat. First class doesn't hurt, either. Yes, I like to look out the window and remain still in Jesus and worship. I will drive if possible, but I need to prepare if I have to fly. And God helps me tolerate it.

Dying is a primary fear with anxiety patients. I take good care of myself, get regular checkups, eat well, exercise, and honor and respect the vessel God gave me. I avoid risky situations; my "thrills" lie in fellowship, ministry, time with friends and family, and shopping. I am grateful for the book of Revelation and the assurance that there is a home after death. But I am human with a family and a purpose. Death is not a desire for me right now. I will trust God with that one.

I have anxiety. I can't do it all or avoid it all. But I embrace my fears with my armor of faith. Knowing anxiety can lurk, I work hard to work through it. And I am at peace with that.

Jodi Howe

Dear Father,

You are my way through anxiety. Please continue to teach me more so wisdom prevails and healing continues. Jesus took His cross and maintains the glory that this sacrifice has brought the world.

Lord, I want to learn to heal through this anxiety, while walking alongside your Son. Thank You for your continued strength.

In Jesus's beautiful name, amen!

Take Aways:

Action Steps:

Night 19

I used to say yes to everything, many times without praying beforehand. I believed that if I was not doing, working, or stressing, I was not living. I was a significant people pleaser.

Where does that nonsense come from? The world! When I started to apply my best yeses to my calendar, my anxiety dropped, and my joy of life began.

 Tip of the night: Protect your schedule.

And on the seventh day God ended His work which He had done, and He rested on the seventh day from all of His work which He had done. Then God blessed the seventh day and sanctified it, because in it He rested from all His work which God had created and made.
Genesis 2:2-3 NKJV

Running at the speed of light every day can be exhausting and overwhelming, taking a toll on your spirit, soul, and body. It's important to slow down and give yourself the rest and recovery you need to maintain your physical and mental well-being.

Respect that you need downtime and rest. It seems so obvious, but human rest is taken for granted.

I am not just talking about sleeping seven to eight hours a night. Resting your mind and spirit is necessary too. I suggest saying "no" more often to events, meetings, or a busy social life that bogs you down. Avoid jam-packing your schedule because you are fearful of letting others down. If they respect you, they should respect your need for rest.

The Air That I Breathe

There are some jobs and careers that only allow a little of this. But if you honor your schedule by prioritizing better, you can find some hidden time to rest and replenish. This may entail less social time with extended friends and family.

You are ineffective towards giving this life, this gift from God, your all if you constantly give yourself to others. Additionally, you are more anxious if you do not honor rest. Even God set an example of this essential part of life.

Father God,

You showed us the importance of rest by setting the example that hard work needs its downtime. The seventh day, the Sabbath, is a commandment I need to follow. Moreover, I need Your help in giving me rest in my mind and life, every day.

In Jesus's name, amen!

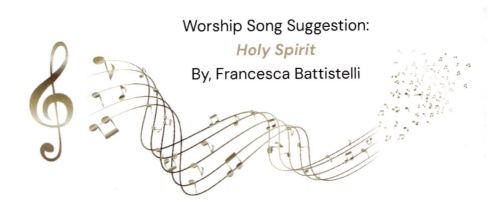

Worship Song Suggestion:
Holy Spirit
By, Francesca Battistelli

Jodi Howe

Take Aways:

Action Steps:

Day 20

I have always been a girly girl, loving makeup, clothes, jewelry, and pretty things. It's how my eyes smile—not idolizing things, but enjoying them.

Beauty is everywhere in the physical realm. But nothing beats a beautiful heart and soul living for Jesus.

 Tip of the day: Beauty is in the eye of the beholder.

Finally, brethren, whatever things are true, whatever things are noble, whatever things are just, whatever things are pure, whatever things are lovely, whatever things are of good report, if there is any virtue and if there is anything praiseworthy—meditate on these things. Philippians 4:8 NKJV

Surround yourself with lovely and positive things.

Along with keeping your mind filled with beautiful thoughts, decorating your home and surroundings with beautiful things helps improve focus and decrease anxiety.

- Art
- Fresh flowers
- Furniture
- Paint colors
- Positive words and inspiration
- Artifacts from your past to promote positive memory

One of my more robust "love languages" is words of affirmation. And nothing is more beautiful than affirming a fellow sister or brother in Christ that they matter, are essential, are acknowledged, and are beautiful.

Jodi Howe

Beauty surrounds us in the physical realm in our children, spouses, friends, and family. Acknowledging the beauty around us is essential in maintaining a positive environment for your mind.

Surrounding yourself with decorative beauty is easier than you think, even on a tight budget. Travel to a rescue mission or thrift store. They always have something beautiful that is no longer needed from another. Remember, someone else's junk can be your treasure!

Dear Father,

Thank You for the beauty You have given us through art, nature, collectibles, décor, people's hearts, and so much more. Beauty can bring such joy, even through sad moments. Whether through a helpful hand or a cherished piece of clay, please remind me more often to search for beauty every day and everywhere.

In Jesus's name, amen!

Take Aways:

Action Steps:

Night 20

As I publish this book, I am going through a divorce and currently facing big struggles. It is not exactly what one would consider a peaceful time. Yet, in the middle of the messes around me, God provides me with a peace that surpasses all understanding. He gives me knowledge and helps me trust that He works everything out for good. Little by little, I can see He is doing that. God is peace. I am a testimony to that.

> *Tip of the night: Peace is not the absence of problems, it's the presence of God.*

Be anxious for nothing, but in everything by prayer and supplication, with thanksgiving, let your requests be made known to God; and the peace of God, which surpasses all understanding, will guard your hearts and mind through Christ Jesus. Philippians 4:6–7 NKJV

A peace that surpasses all understanding! In other words, God provides general peace when we pray to Him. A peace the world can't understand, because the world rallies around being anxious, worrisome, and fearful.

He is the God of peace. Merciful, graceful, a way maker, and a miracle worker. And this peace? It's possible and livable. When you are in the presence of God, this all-surpassing peace will calm you in a storm, center you in a crisis, and hold you in grief.

I hope you know this peace.

Father God,

I need this peace. I desire this peace. I ask You for this peace. I am so grateful to You for healing me from anxiety. Please keep guiding me on this

The Air That I Breathe

pathway to peace and transformation of spirit. Please protect my heart and fuel my thoughts that only glorify You.

Thank You for Your son, Christ Jesus. amen.

Worship Song Suggestion:
PEACE
By, We The Kingdom,
Bethel Music

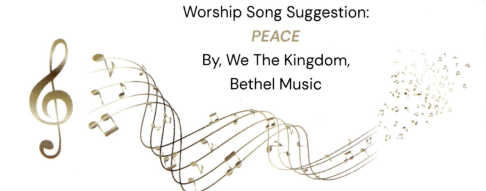

Take Aways:

___

Action Steps:

Day 21

*I*was the class clown in grade school. True story. I've always loved comedy, and growing up in an Italian household was comedy in itself. My holidays were filled with family laughing around the dinner tables, cousins teasing each other, siblings joking and laughing. It makes me smile just thinking about the fun we had growing up.

I will choose laughter over any other emotion, anytime. And wow, how it makes you feel. It's sent from God.

Tip of the day: Laughter is the best medicine.

Then our mouth was filled with laughter, and our tongue with singing. Then they said among the nations, "The Lord has done great things for them." The Lord has done great things for us, And we are glad." Psalms 126:2–3 NKJV

Of course, God has a sense of humor. Yes, He encourages laughter. With all of Jesus's intense work on earth, there is no doubt he had many reasons to laugh with joy through His journeys and teachings.

Speaking of laughter, joy comes hand in hand. And in this complicated world, there is plenty to laugh at lovingly. Studies show that laughter can reduce anxiety. The act of laughing is like deep breathing in its ability to increase the oxygen in our bodies. Coupled with reducing stress hormones, the increased oxygen in the body helps lead to muscle relaxation. By laughing, we reduce the physical symptoms of anxiety.

Watch a comedy show or funny movie, find a clean comedian online, hang around fun-loving people, and always laugh till you cry tears of joy for Jesus. Because, after all, Jesus is joy!

Jodi Howe

Dear God,

Laughter is a medicinal cure, and I thank You for its potency and therapeutic nature. I ask You for a forever joyful and amusing heart to offset life's complicated nature.

With a gleeful smile, I honor Jesus's name. amen!

The Air That I Breathe

Take Aways:

Action Steps:

Night 21

I'll never forget a few years back in a Bible study; a woman had a complex story she was living through. She would share it for prayer requests but complain about it in a way that demonstrated she was always looking for someone to blame.

I was a new Christian who only knew a few Scriptures. Proverbs 3:5-6 was my most memorized one. So, during one of her "woah is me" sessions, I sternly reminded her that this "trust" is not 99.44%. It's 100%.

She didn't like hearing what I said. And there was tension in the room.

The Lord humbled me years later with that same resistance of pure trust.

Yet today, I still stand on that premise. I am living this right now. A complete and absolute trust that God will set my path straight. There is no wiggle room for this.

 Tip of the night: Trust.

Trust in the LORD with all your heart, and lean not on your understanding; In all your ways acknowledge Him, And He shall direct your paths. Proverbs 3:5-6 NKJV

I am convinced this Scripture was written just for me. But seriously, besides the "The Lord's Prayer," this one sums it up! That alone should give you peace, knowing that this, too, shall pass. Trust with all your heart that God has got your anxiety. No doubt! Yes, He hears you, sees you, and is healing you. Stop letting negative thoughts tell you otherwise. Life, people, the internet, and the world will tell you that God is a mythical figure incapable of miracles. But take note: Jesus

The Air That I Breathe

conquered the world on the cross. He is a loving, "real God" with love for His children and empathy for their pain. Talk to God, cry to God, wrestle with Him, plea to Him, and love Him. He wants you to give your anxiety to Him. And then, only then, will you see a more straightforward pathway to peace. I am the testimony to this.

Father God,

This is my prayer in every breathe that I take. Please help me commit this Scripture to memory so that when fear, doubt, and mental pain creep in, I can overpower it with these God-breathed words.

In Jesus's precious name. amen!

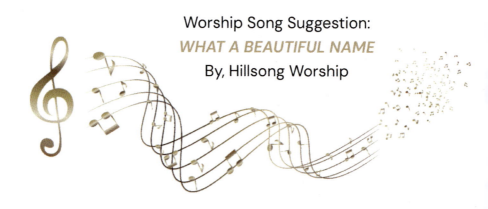

Worship Song Suggestion:
WHAT A BEAUTIFUL NAME
By, Hillsong Worship

Jodi Howe

Take Aways:

Action Steps:

Day 22

This book is how I am turning all I've been through with anxiety over to God and His glory. While suffering through the healing stages, I looked for a book like this. I needed advice. I was seeking God. I didn't want just a story of redemption from anxiety; I desperately needed daily hope to teach me tried and true tips to apply every day so I could begin to feel better again.

I took notes of all the things I experienced and wrote this book.

It has been over six years in the making, rewriting, and praying, and now God's timing has become clear that it is ready for publication. Praise Jesus.

Tip of the day: Turn your pain into power.

I will instruct you and teach you in the way you should go; I will guide you with My eye. Psalms 32:8 NKJV

Your anxiety is not a result of bad luck. It's not a curse from bad behavior or actions. It's not the wrath of God. But it may be your current health concern. And you can help lower the stigma by acknowledging it and discussing it more, whether to a doctor, a friend, a group, a pastor, or other trusted authority. Mental illness is a stigma that we (as sufferers) need to lower. And that begins by starting the conversation.

Learning to live with mental health problems is made more difficult when someone experiences prejudice caused by stigma. Stigma can be used to exclude and marginalize people. The bias and fear caused by stigma may even prevent people from coming forward and seeking the help they need.

When I was diagnosed, I was petrified to tell anyone. That stigma was hovering over like a blackened cloud, ready to burst into a storm. What would people think? Would they mock or ask me to get over it? Would they end relationships with me, labeling me crazy?

When I finally shared my testimony with some moms at a playdate, they all came forward with their testimonies of depression, anxiety, unhappiness, and stress; in other words, they were humans experiencing *life*.

And for the first time, I didn't feel alone or misunderstood.

Then, my transparency and open-book philosophy took a different turn, encouraging me to share this with you. My final major bout with anxiety opened a new world in Jesus Christ. He provided healing that I never could have imagined. Through His counsel and love, I can share this comeback as a testimony to that love through this book.

Dear God,

I am grateful for Your wisdom as it brings me hope. I know I can sail through any storm, big or small, with you. As I learn to praise you in my storms, I will eventually dance in the rain and lift my hands in joy, praising You. When I witness the sun creeping over the rainbow, I am reminded of your miraculous promise of Jesus's return. You are a good, good father.

Through Jesus's name, I pray this to you, amen.

Take Aways:

Action Steps:

Night 22

I pray you are feeling better. I pray you are in His Word. I pray you are seeking God more.

You can do all things through Christ who strengthens you.

> *Tip of the night: Love the Lord God with all your heart, all your soul, and all your mind.*

And now abide faith, hope, love, these three; but the greatest of these is love. 1 Corinthians 13:13 NKJV

Continue to pray, learn, trust–live in faith, hope, and, most importantly, love.

I couldn't, in good faith, write a book that did not speak to or honor or glorify the Lord Jesus Christ. Why? He is the reason I can write this.

The Lord Jesus Christ saved my life. The least I can do is help others find that peace.

Unlike depression, anxiety gives us a tremendous fear of dying. It gives us a jittery, non-peaceful-like predisposition. It's a worrisome, fearful existence that is the polar opposite of who God is. God is the God of peace, who makes a way when it seems there is no other way.

It wasn't until I learned about the power of the Holy Spirit and a relationship with Jesus that I felt peace through the mental storms of life.

My anxiety started in my young adult life, significantly interfering with my plans.

But I can see now that God was always there knocking on my door; it was a matter of my willingness to answer it!

Friends, accepting God's plan for my life is where my "fearless living" began and continues to flourish spiritually with daily hope.

I used to think anxiety was my cross to bear, but I learned that Jesus had already paid for that cross at Calvary. I began to feel empowered about how He could see me through anxiety and work through all of my life's mental storms and challenges.

Life is hard, and we do hard things. Sometimes, we have to walk through the valley of the shadow of death. But God promises us specifically in Philippians 4:13, "I can do all things through Christ who strengthens me."

This newfound revelation allows this secular proverb to speak volumes in my life: "It is truly not what happens to us in life; it is how we allow God to handle it."

The power of Scripture, like in Proverbs 3:5-6, explains *how* we handle it. When we consider changing our worldview towards God's view, we learn to respect the Spirit He left for us to lean on. We divinely yearn to start transforming our minds to be more like Him because we are not meant to do this life alone.

Trusting in the Lord, not the world, allows Him to set our paths straight.

God starts to work in us so we can be the brothers or sisters to all who need hope for today and always.

His power provides healing through hardships of life.

His presence is the peace through the mental storms.

His wisdom offers solutions to problems and a keen direction from confusion.

His love is the opposite of pain, loss, fear and doubt.

Jodi Howe

*Jesus
is the way,
the truth,
And the life!*

2 Corinthians 12:9 (my paraphrase) says, "His grace is sufficient for you today; His power is made perfect in weakness."

Father God,

I love You for all You have sacrificed, taught me, tested me, believed in me, and inevitably blessed me with. I am forever grateful. Please continue to remind me of Your greatest gifts. Instill in me the faith and belief in You and Your wonders. Grant hope for my healing and peaceful existence. Thank You for Your everlasting love.

It's in Jesus's name that is love. amen!

Worship Song Suggestion:
GOODNESS OF GOD
By, CeCe Winans

and

Worship Song Suggestion:
GRATITUDE
By, Brandon Lake

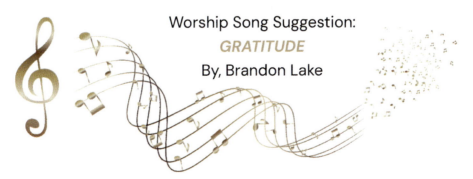

Take Aways:

Action Steps:

22 Day Reflection

> *Acceptance doesn't mean resignation; it means understanding that something is what it is and there's got to be a way through it.*
> *-Michael J. Fox*

1. What skills have you developed to manage and accept anxiety as your health concern?

   _____
   _____

2. How is understanding and utilizing the Holy Spirit becoming a game-changer in conquering your fears?

   _____
   _____

Take a few minutes and journal about how you are becoming a "new creation" in God and how it has impacted your approach to anxiety.

_____
_____
_____

The Air That I Breathe

Altar Call

God's love is unconditional and all-encompassing. He loves us no matter what we do or how we feel. He is always there for us, even when we are anxious or overwhelmed. He understands our struggles and is willing to help us through them. He can provide us with peace and comfort in times of distress. He can also give us strength and courage to face our fears and anxieties. God's love is a powerful source of hope and healing and can help us.

Can I offer you a tried and true prayer through an altar call to start this journey?

If you can, play this on a music streaming app.

Prayer Song Suggestion:

GRATITUD-Instrumental

Colectivo1 – Roberto Bautista

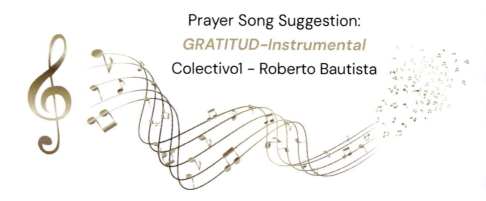

Jodi Howe

My Commitment

Father God of the Universe,

Your name is holy and powerful. Thank You for promising me a home in heaven and a savior to help me walk this earth. Thank You for all you have done and will continue to provide me with the bread of life. Forgive me for my sins and teach me to forgive others who have harmed me. Lead me from the world's temptations and protect me from the enemy who tries to attack me. I ask for Jesus to come into my heart right now. At this moment, I commit my life to You through His blood and His holy body.

Amen.

I committed my life to Jesus Christ.

Day _____

Time _____

TIP of the Day

Tip of the day: Take a leap of faith	13
Tip of the day: Doctor, doctor. Give me the news …	21
Tip of the day: Don't instigate your anxiety!	27
Tip of the day: "A" is for anxiety.	33
Tip of the day: The air that I breathe.	38
Tip of the day: Give your first five minutes to God.	44
Tip of the day: Get movin'!	48
Tip of the day: An apple a day may keep anxiety away.	57
Tip of the day: Mind over matter.	62
Tip of the day: Rely while you occupy.	68
Tip of the day: Acceptance is not defeat when you understand anxiety's relevance as a part of life.	74
Tip of the day: Anxiety does not discriminate.	80
Tip of the day: April showers bring May flowers.	86
Tip of the day: Here is a breathe of fresh air.	92
Tip of the day: Day planner.	99
Tip of the day: Tidy up your mind.	104
Tip of the day: Take a day trip.	109
Tip of the day: Milestones are life markers, not fear factors.	115
Tip of the day: Flex on the power of the Holy Spirit.	121
Tip of the day: Beauty is in the eye of the beholder.	128
Tip of the day: Laughter is the best medicine.	134
Tip of the day: Turn your pain into power.	140

TIP of the Night

Tip of the night: This too shall pass!	16
Tip of the night: God gave us modern medicine.	24
Tip of the night: Prayer is the bridge between panic and peace.	30
Tip of the night: ♪ Don't worry, be holy. ♪	35
Tip of the night: Make tonight a "spa" ritual night!	41
Tip of the night: Jot it down!	45
Tip of the night: Raise a hallelujah!	51
Tip of the night: Consume the Holy Spirit.	59
Tip of the night: He is God; you are not!	65
Tip of the night: Heaven's hydration.	71
Tip of the night: Give it to God and go to sleep.	77
Tip of the night: Use your "wise mind" to rid your crazy thoughts.	83
Tip of the night: Love can move mountains.	89
Tip of the night: Be generous and pray for others tonight!	94
Tip of the night: Plant yourself to sleep!	101
Tip of the night: Filter your feelings.	106
Tip of the night: How to find your spiritual REM.	112
Tip of the night: Technically speaking ...	118
Tip of the night: Protect your schedule.	125
Tip of the night: Peace is not the absence of problems, it's the presence of God.	131
Tip of the night: Trust.	137
Tip of the night: Love the Lord God with all your heart, all your soul, and all your mind.	143

ABOUT THE AUTHOR

Jodi Howe is an author and award-winning podcaster of the show, The Air That I Breathe. She is also a speaker and emcee who loves to write blogs and prayers to encourage Kingdom living. Her love for music and how it touches the soul keeps her in the music industry as it has for decades. She serves on her church's worship team and is a vocal coach.

Jodi is a mother to two children and a lazy cat. They reside in Cary, North Carolina. Please connect with Jodi on her website, www.jodihowe.com.

With all my Gratitude

Thank you, Andrea Lende, for your tireless support and direction in publishing to get this in the right hands and hearts.

Thank you, Misty Phillip, for being my loyal, godly sister and cheerleader of "all the things" in ministry. This book is a big "Eek!"

To my dear Abby and Moro, you are so precious to me.

Thank you, Mom and Dad, for loving me and supporting my creative talents.

I love you all!

Made in the USA
Middletown, DE
27 November 2023